Invasive Medical Skills

A Multimedia Approach

By

Mark Stoneham

and

Jon Westbrook

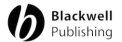

Blackwell
Publishing

Published by Blackwell Publishing
Blackwell Publishing, Inc., 350 Main Street, Malden, Massachusetts 02148-5020, USA
Blackwell Publishing Ltd, 9600 Garsington Road, Oxford OX4 2DQ, UK
Blackwell Publishing Asia Pty Ltd, 550 Swanston Street, Carlton, Victoria 3053, Australia

First published

1   2007

Library of Congress Cataloging-in-Publication Data

Stoneham, Mark.
   Invasive medical skills : a multimedia approach / by Mark Stoneham and Jon
Westbrook.
          p. ; cm.
   Includes bibliographical references and index.
   ISBN-13: 978-1-4051-5986-9 (alk. paper)
   ISBN-10: 1-4051-5986-3 (alk. paper)
   1.   Therapeutics. 2.   Surgery, Operative. I. Westbrook, Jon. II. Title.
   [DNLM: 1.   Catheterization—methods—Handbooks. 2.   Intubation—methods—
Handbooks. 3.   Punctures—methods—Handbooks. WB 39 S878i 2007]

   RM103.S76 2007
   615.5'3—dc22

                                                                        2007019937

ISBN: 978-1-4051-5986-9

A catalogue record for this title is available from the British Library

Set in 9/12 Trebuchet by Charon Tec Ltd (A Macmillan Company), Chennai, India
www.charontec.com
Printed and bound in Singapore by Fabulous Printers Pte Ltd

Commissioning Editors: Martin Sugden and Vicki Noyes
Editorial Assistants: Ellie Bonnet and Robin Harries
Development Editor: Beckie Brand
Production Controller: Debbie Wyer
DVD produced by: Meg Barton and Emantras

For further information on Blackwell Publishing, visit our website:
http://www.blackwellpublishing.com

Contents

DVD: Installation

This DVD-ROM should start automatically upon insertion.

Alternatively, or to restore after quitting, browse the DVD and double click the file 'SW_Win.exe' (if using Windows 2000 or higher) or 'SW_Mac.exe' (if using Mac OS 10.0 or higher). Please double click the application to run.

Please note that this DVD-ROM is not designed for use in standalone DVD players.

Minimum technical requirements
OS : Windows 2000 or higher / Mac 10.0 or higher
Resolution : 1024 × 768 pixels
Flash Player : 8.0 or higher
RAM Size : 256 MB RAM or higher

DVD Contents

Every chapter in the book is supported by the following features on the DVD

Videoclips

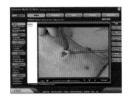

- Demonstrating every procedure
- Including an audio commentary

Animations

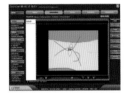

- Showing what is going on under the skin during each of these procedures
- Showing how complications can occur and what to do about them

Notes

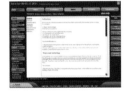

- Detailing each procedure
- Indications – contraindications – theory and technology – tricks of the trade – complications – references

Anatomy

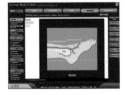

- Drawings, photos, or surface anatomy
- Including a 'show/hide labels' feature

Equipment

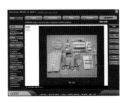

- Photos of each item of equipment needed for each procedure
- Including a 'show/hide labels' feature

From Our Medical Student Reviewers

The DVD was reviewed by a selection of newly qualified junior doctors:

"This is a really good idea and use of a multimedia resource. The videos are especially good… All the procedures listed are relevant for F1 and will provide reassurance for a doctor who is just starting and probably has not performed some of these for a while."

"This is an excellent idea – I love it. I think the idea of having an animation as well as a video demonstration is fantastic. I also like the fact that you've included the anatomy as well… I think the thing that makes this a good idea is the fact that you've linked the videos with animations, anatomy and notes. I think the topics covered are excellent and would have been useful for me as a medical student and also now as I am about to start work as a junior doctor."

"I wish that there had been a similar resource available for me. To be honest, this would still be massively useful for me now and for a few years to come I imagine. The DVD section is clearly laid out, the video sections are very good and give a clear indication of procedure… I think this is a really good idea and I see it being very useful not only in medical education but also for individual use."

"I think that the content for each available entry is excellent. The videos are clear and instructive. The animations are a helpful addendum. The notes, and in particular the sections on complications of the procedure are outstanding and this information is often difficult to find elsewhere. I particularly like the fact that there is an included section on anatomy for each clinical skill, with clear photographs and labels. I have looked for this kind of information before and it was very difficult to find!"

"… this resource would be invaluable as a junior doctor. It is often quite difficult to learn clinical skills as you have to see the procedure at least once before you are allowed to try yourself! For some of the rarer procedures it can be very difficult to even see one let alone practise yourself. [It] allows students and doctors to observe the procedures in the 'ideal' situation before practising on the clinical skills dummies we have in the hospital."

About the Authors

Mark Stoneham, MA, FRCA, is Consultant Anaesthetist at the John Radcliffe Hospital, Oxford and Honorary Senior Clinical Lecturer at Oxford University. He spent 5 years in the Royal Navy and Royal Marines, received anaesthetic training in the South West and Ann Arbor, Michigan. His clinical and research interests are in regional and vascular anaesthesia.

Jon Westbrook, MRCP, FRCA, is Consultant Anaesthetist at the John Radcliffe Hospital, Oxford and Honorary Senior Clinical Lecturer at Oxford University. He trained in general medicine before commencing his anaesthetic training in Oxford and the University of Maryland in Baltimore. His clinical sub-specialty interests are in neuro-anaesthesia and neuro-intensive care.

Introduction

This project was conceived whilst watching medical students and trainee doctors struggling to gain competence and confidence with a myriad of invasive medical procedures. This reinforced our own memories of the stress and anxiety associated with learning new procedures. When things are getting difficult, a busy hospital can feel like a very lonely place.

Patients have had to endure multiple attempts at venesection and arterial blood gas sampling. They have undergone lumbar punctures in which they were almost nailed to the wall with the spinal needle and suffered a chest drain insertion after a routine central line placement. This is not to mention the trainee's own fear, embarrassment and escalating tremor, as they move from one failed procedure to another.

The old adage of 'see one, do one, teach one' is no longer acceptable in an era of reduced training hours and competency-based assessment. If the one you see is not done well, then nor is the one you do and nor will be the one you teach. So mistakes and bad practice sustain themselves. Much better to learn from other clinicians' experience and their mistakes, as well as the tricks they have learnt along the way to avoid problems and to get out of trouble when needed. The real benefactors of this support for your learning will be your patients.

By pulling together all the important clinical techniques with video that you can watch, when you like, as many times as you like, you will be able to embark on even new procedures with confidence and competence. Your practice will also be enhanced by greater background knowledge of the important principles of areas such as sterile technique, sedation and the effective use of local anaesthesia.

We do not pretend that the techniques shown are the only ones, nor necessarily the best. For some procedures there are almost as many techniques as there are clinicians doing them. However the authors have successfully used these methods for a combined experience of over 40 years of busy clinical practice and by following the guidance given you can fast-track through to a level of competence for which your patients will only thank you.

There are some procedures which even busy clinicians will only rarely see or do: needle cricothyroidotomy, tension pneumothorax or venous cutdown, for example. Yet these are the very procedures that can save lives. To embark on one of these with only the memory of dry words on a page read 10 years ago is enough to give anyone palpitations. With the benefit of watching these videos you are more likely to do the right thing at the right time and do it well without being paralysed by fear.

There are few things more miserable than inflicting pain on a patient and failing to achieve what you set out to do. There are few things more satisfying than doing an invasive medical procedure, painlessly and well for a grateful patient. You do not need to endure medical procedures – learn to do them properly and you will enjoy them. Good luck.

I
Venous
Section

I Venous

II Arterial

III Central Venous

IV Airway

V Thoracic

VI Others

VII Supplemental Skills

1. Venous Cannulation

If the area where you intend to insert a cannula is hairy, gently shave the skin first with a razor.

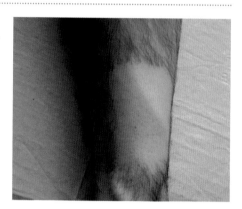

- You will see the veins better.
- It will make the cannulation easier.
- The dressing will stick better.
- It will hurt the patient less when the dressing is removed.

Apply a tourniquet and identify a suitable vein.

- A colleague squeezing the arm or a rubber glove will suffice in the absence of a tourniquet.
- Tourniquet pressure should be above venous but below arterial pressure so that the veins fill.
- Try not to snag hairs with the rubber glove, it hurts!
- Reusable tourniquets may be an infection risk.
- Make gravity work for you: dangle the arm down by the side and kneel down beside the patient.
- Tap the vein with the back of your hand, this releases nitric oxide into the vein wall causing vasodilatation.
- Difficult veins need patience; if you know where to find them they may be palpable even when invisible.

Prep the skin before infiltrating the intended puncture site with local anaesthetic.

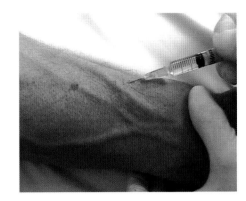

- Allow the alcohol to evaporate before inserting a needle, otherwise it will sting. This is also necessary for antisepsis.
- Local anaesthetic is required for any cannula larger than 20G (pink). People who claim that local hurts more than the cannula or makes cannulation more difficult are wrong.

Applying counter traction with your non-dominant hand, puncture the skin and then align the cannula with the vein before advancing along the vessel at least 1–2 mm.

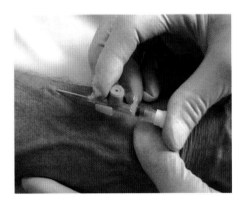

- Aim to pierce the skin with the first movement, and then puncture the vein with a second action. These two elements may occur simultaneously, but they do not have to.
- The veins in elderly patients tend to be very mobile. Once you are through the skin, you need to immobilise the vein using counter-traction. You may require a rapid 'stabbing motion' to puncture the vein, which will otherwise run away from the needle!

Once blood is seen in the chamber, withdraw the needle until you see blood tracking up the cannula, then advance the cannula along the vein. Now, release the tourniquet.

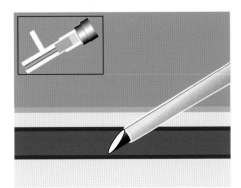

- Remember don't withdraw the needle until the cannula itself is in the vein.
- Avoid touching the cannula itself which is sterile.
- If you meet resistance it may be a venous valve. Gently realign the needle and try to advance it further. Alternatively, attach a syringe of saline to the cannula and advance it whilst flushing with saline.

I Venous   II Arterial   III Central Venous   IV Airway   V Thoracic   VI Others   VII Supplemental Skills

Remove the needle whilst occluding the vein and immediately cap the cannula.

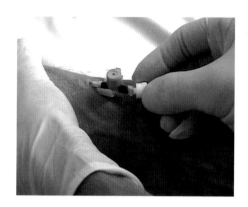

- Allow blood to fill the cannula before you cap it to avoid air embolism. Whilst this is a good practice in adults, it is also essential in paediatrics.

After applying a dressing, flush the cannula with saline solution.

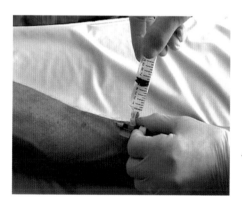

- Carefully examine and/or palpate the site during injection to confirm correct placement. Any resistance, pain or swelling suggests that the cannula is not in the vein.
- Always flush a cannula with saline prior to an injection to confirm that it has not tissued.
- Always suspect and exclude accidental arterial placement of a venous cannula – particularly, if you do not site the cannula yourself – and, especially, if the cannula is sited in the antecubital fossa.

If you get initial flashback of blood as you pass the needle the first time, but then do not get flashback of blood when you withdraw the needle, all is not necessarily lost. The situation may be rescued with care.

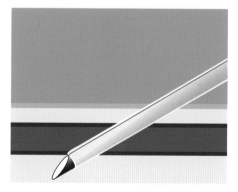

- The most likely cause is that you have punctured the back wall of the vein and have now transfixed the vein with your needle.

Keeping the tourniquet applied, withdraw the needle until you can see the lumen of the cannula.

- This enables you to see when blood enters the cannula.

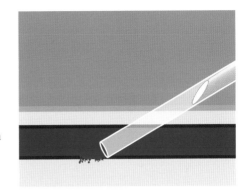

Maintaining counter traction with your non-dominant hand, withdraw the cannula and needle with the other hand as slowly as possible until you see a flashback of blood.

- The flashback occurs as the cannula tip once again re-enters the vein lumen.

Now, all in one motion, advance the cannula and needle together into the vein. Then remove the needle and secure the Luer lock cap

- Flush the cannula with saline to confirm intravenous placement.
- With practice, this technique will succeed more often than not.
- Other possible causes of failure include:
  - Missing the vein altogether, in which case you should start all over again
  - A valve within the vein – this is usually not recoverable unless you can push the needle through the valve to the other side – often the cannula will go through the wall of the vein instead
  - Thrombosis or obliteration of the vein caused by previous cannulation.

Do not re-insert the needle into the cannula during repeated attempts at venous cannulation.

- You can shear the tip off the cannula which could embolise into the patient.

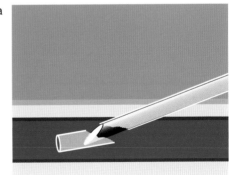

Always dispose of sharps carefully to avoid needlestick:

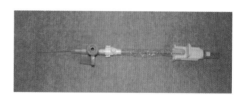

- Never re-sheath a needle.
- IV cannulae are now available with safety mechanisms to reduce the incidence of needlestick.

2. Putting Up a Drip

Check the intended intravenous solution including the contents and expiry date.

- Consider whether the contents are appropriate for this patient, particularly the electrolytes, sugar contents and osmolarity. For example, 0.9% normal saline contains 154 mmol sodium per litre – very few patients need fluids containing this amount of sodium continuously.

Remove all packaging and caps. Insert the giving set spike into the connection port.

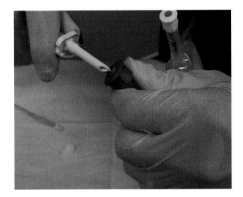

- A twisting motion will get the spike through the rubber bung.
- Do not touch the spike or rubber bung with your hands, they are sterile.
- Take care not to push the spike through the side wall of the tubing which will then leak.

With the bag and giving set inverted, squeeze the bag to fill the chambers.

When the second drip chamber is half full, close the roller valve and turn the set the right way up. Now run through the giving set to exclude all air.

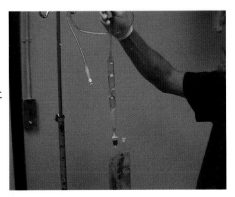

- Put the end over a sink or waste bin so that neither you nor the floor gets soaked.

I Venous   II Arterial   III Central Venous   IV Airway   V Thoracic   VI Others   VII Supplemental Skills

Connect to the IV cannula by gently compressing the vein, removing the cap and firmly screwing on the Luer lock connection.

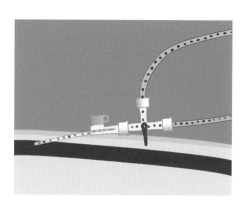

- Occluding the vein during connection requires gentle pressure over the vein proximal to the end of the cannula. If you compress over the cannula itself, blood may still leak out.

- Consider whether you need a three-way tap as an additional injection port.

- If you do use a three-way tap, avoid giving two different drugs through it – it is possible to give a large bolus of one drug if the cannula becomes blocked or turned off.

Commence the IV and check the flow rate.

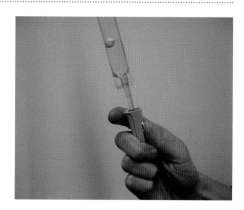

- As a ballpark figure, 1 drop per second is approximately 120 ml per hour – this is an '8 hourly bag' of fluid.

3. Venesection

Apply the tourniquet and ask the patient to open and close their fist whilst you gently tap the veins.

- Tap the vein with the back of your hand – this releases nitric oxide into the vein wall causing vasodilatation.
- Think which blood samples you need to take. Get all the bottles and calculate how much blood you will need.
- Even better, think what bloods are required the day before and get the phlebotomists to take the blood for you!
- Take your time at all stages – everybody gets stressed – particularly you – when you miss and have to stick the patient again.

Prep the skin.

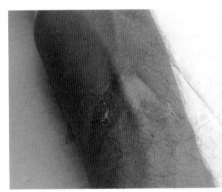

- Needles hurt! A needle-phobic patient can be a real challenge. You can make patients (particularly children) needle-phobic if you allow things to get out of hand.
- Local anaesthetic creams (EMLA or amethocaine) can make a big difference provided they are given time to work (at least 20 min).
- Alternately, ethyl chloride spray will give you immediate cryo-analgesia lasting for a few seconds.
- So-called 'Painless Venepuncture' without EMLA or amethocaine is also possible.

You must be able to hold the syringe absolutely steady whilst aspirating blood, this takes practice.

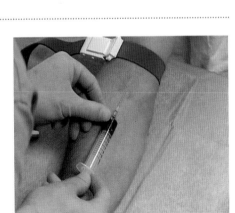

- Hold the syringe so that you do not need to change your grip between venepuncture and commencing the aspiration of blood.

I Venous   II Arterial   III Central Venous   IV Airway   V Thoracic   VI Others   VII Supplemental Skills

Select your puncture site and pass the needle rapidly and smoothly into the lumen of the vessel.

- Use a green (18G) needle – haemolysis can result if you draw blood up through a very fine needle.

- The trickiest bit occurs after you have successfully entered the vein. Be patient – the vein has to refill as you aspirate – so do not rush – you will only collapse the vein and risk puncturing the back wall with the needle.

- Brace your hand against the patient to keep your hands steady during the aspiration of blood. This takes patience and practice.

- The Vacutainer system makes this easier but you must still keep your hand *absolutely* still whilst blood is being aspirated.

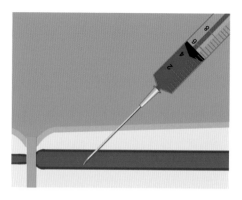

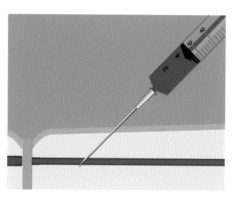

When venesection is complete release the tourniquet. Place a dry cotton ball over the puncture site and rapidly withdraw the needle. Apply pressure for 2–3 min to prevent a haematoma developing.

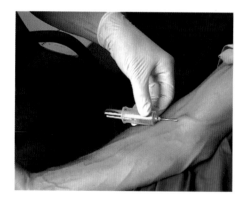

Transfer the blood to a suitable container taking care to avoid needlestick injury.

- *Never* re-sheath a used needle. You *will* eventually stick yourself doing this.

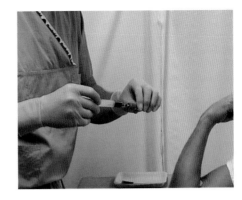

Place the needle directly into a sharps bin and label the bottle immediately at the patient's side.

- Most haematology/biochemistry departments have non-negotiable rules regarding the labelling of samples – they cannot be labelled retrospectively – so get it right first time to prevent having to take the whole sample again.

I Venous   II Arterial   III Central Venous   IV Airway   V Thoracic   VI Others   VII Supplemental Skills

I Venous   II Arterial   III Central Venous   IV Airway   V Thoracic   VI Others   VII Supplemental Skills

4. Femoral Stab

Prep the skin thoroughly with antiseptic solution as this is a potentially contaminated area.

- Chlorhexidine or betadine is appropriate.
- Remember the antiseptic has to dry before it is effective.

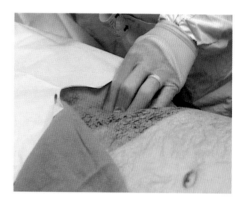

Palpate the femoral arterial pulse just below the inguinal ligament. The femoral vein lies medial to the artery.

- The NAVY acronym (Nerve – Artery – Vein – Y-fronts) is useful here – going from lateral to medial along the inguinal ligament.
- Alternatively the 'V-A-N' goes up the inguinal ligament from medial to lateral.

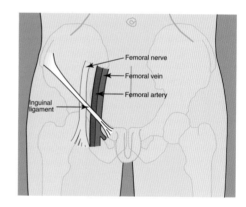

Femoral nerve
Femoral vein
Femoral artery
Inguinal ligament

Infiltrate the skin and underlying tissues with local anaesthetic.

● Whilst adequate analgesia is important, puncturing the femoral vein with the local anaesthetic needle should be avoided. Therefore, do not go too deep with your local anaesthetic needle.

Direct the needle towards the femoral vein aspirating as you advance. On entering the vessel steady your hand and aspirate the required amount of blood.

● It is sometimes difficult to remain steady in these circumstances. Use one hand to stabilise the needle whilst the other (usually your dominant hand) aspirates the blood.

● If you accidentally puncture the femoral artery do not worry, you can still aspirate the blood required but then you must maintain pressure for at least 5 min afterwards to avoid a haematoma.

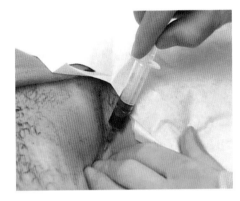

On completion rapidly withdraw the needle and apply pressure for at least 3 min.

● This time should be longer if the patient is coagulopathic.

Meanwhile you or your assistant should transfer the blood to the relevant bottles.

● Label the bottles immediately – hospital pathology departments usually have non-negotiable rules about the formal identification of laboratory specimens. Failure to comply usually means having to take the sample again!

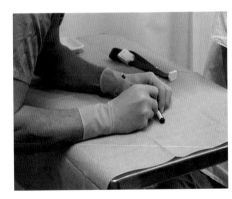

5. Intravenous Injection

Caution is needed injecting drugs directly through a needle.

- The needle can be misplaced very easily with resulting extravasation of the drug.
- If there is an adverse reaction to the injected drug there is limited access for administration of corrective drugs if required.
- If you need to give more than one injection, insert an IV cannula.

Check the ampoule of the drug you are intending to inject including: contents, dose, and expiry date. Draw it up into the syringe and label it.

- Avoid administering drugs which you have not drawn up yourself – if you do have to then *always* check the contents and expiry date of the ampoule yourself.

Apply a tourniquet and identify a suitable vein. This will most often be in the antecubital fossa.

- Take your time.
- Use gravity to help fill the veins.
- Pressure applied by tourniquet, rubber glove or an assistant should be above venous pressure but below arterial to fill the veins.
- Be aware of the underlying brachial artery – inadvertent arterial injection of some drugs is potentially very dangerous.

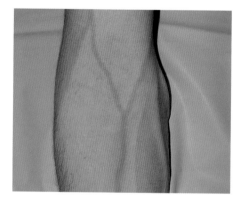

I Venous   II Arterial   III Central Venous   IV Airway   V Thoracic   VI Others   VII Supplemental Skills

Prep the skin with an alcoholic wipe.

- Tap the vein with the back of your hand – this releases nitric oxide into the vein wall causing vasodilatation.

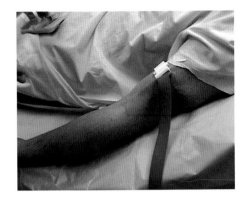

Puncture the vein using the same technique as for venesection.

- Brace your hand against the patient to keep it absolutely still.

Aspirate a little blood to confirm venous placement and then release the tourniquet.

- Ask an assistant to do this or use your non-dominant hand, but be careful not to move the needle in the vein during this manoeuvre.

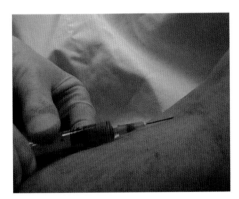

Slowly inject the drug monitoring the patient for any adverse reaction.

Finally apply a cotton wool ball and rapidly withdraw the needle. Maintain firm pressure for at least 3 min.

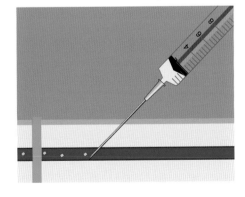

I Venous   II Arterial   III Central Venous   IV Airway   V Thoracic   VI Others   VII Supplemental Skills

6. Intramuscular Injection

Draw up the drugs before you start.

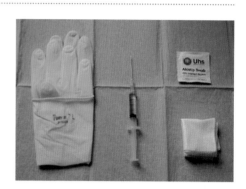

- Avoid administering drugs which you have not drawn up yourself – if you do have to then *always* check the contents and expiry date of the ampoule yourself.

Select a suitable injection site:

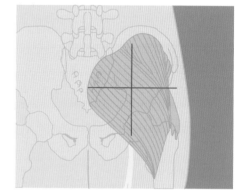

- The choice of site should take into consideration the patient's general physical status and age, and the amount of drug to be given. Assess muscle mass in elderly, thin or cachectic patients.
- Inspect the proposed injection site for signs of inflammation, swelling and infection. Avoid obvious skin lesions.
- There are five suitable IM injection sites:
  1. The upper arm (deltoid) – used for vaccines such as hepatitis B and tetanus toxoid.
  2. The dorsogluteal buttock (gluteus maximus).
  3. The ventrogluteal buttock (gluteus medius).
  4. The vastus lateralis (quadriceps femoris) on the outer side of the femur.
  5. The rectus femoris (anterior quadriceps) – easily accessed for self-administration, or for infants.
- For repeated IM injections, rotate injection sites and document this – this reduces pain and minimises the possibility of muscle atrophy or sterile abscesses.

I Venous   II Arterial   III Central Venous   IV Airway   V Thoracic   VI Others   VII Supplemental Skills

Prep the skin with an alcohol swab and allow the skin to dry.

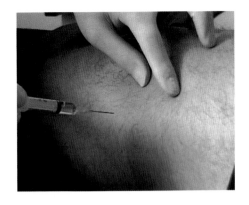

- Allowing the skin to dry before the injection is bacteriocidal as well as reducing the pain of injection.

Gently pull the skin laterally, then insert the needle rapidly in one motion.

- Use the Z-track technique, now recommended for all IM medications. It reduces pain and the incidence of leakage. The lateral skin movement moves the cutaneous and subcutaneous tissues approximately 1-2 cm. After injection, the tissues close over the medication deposit, preventing leakage.
- Remember that moving the skin may distract you from the intended needle destination. Therefore, visualise the underlying muscle that is to receive the injection, and aim for that location, rather than a distinguishing mark on the skin.

Aspirate to exclude intravascular placement then slowly inject the drug.

- Stabilise the needle and syringe with the non-dominant hand before aspirating. This will help reduce needle-tip movement.
- If you aspirate blood, withdraw the needle and start over with fresh medication and a new syringe/needle.

Remove the needle, apply pressure and observe for any adverse reaction.

- Check the site 2-4 h after the injection to ensure there has been no adverse reaction.

I Venous   II Arterial   III Central Venous   IV Airway   V Thoracic   VI Others   VII Supplemental Skills

7. Intradermal Injection

Draw up the drugs first.

- Avoid administering drugs which you have not drawn up yourself – if you do have to then *always* check the contents and expiry date of the ampoule yourself.

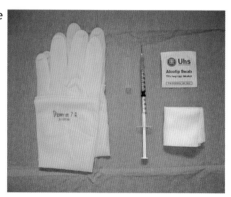

Select a suitable injection site.

- Sites suitable for intradermal testing are similar to those for subcutaneous injections but also include the inner forearm and shoulder blades.
- If it is being used for allergen testing, the area should be labelled indicating the antigen so that an allergic response can be monitored after a specified time lapse.

Prep the skin with an alcohol swab, then allow it to dry.

- Allowing the skin to dry before the injection is bacteriocidal as well as reducing the pain of injection.

Use a 25G or 27G needle inserted at a 10-15° angle into the epidermis.

- Do not aspirate before injection.
- Up to 0.5 ml is injected until a white wheal appears on the skin surface. This often has the appearance of orange peel hence the term 'peau d'orange'.

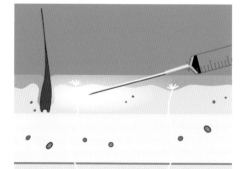

Slowly inject the drug then remove the
needle rapidly.

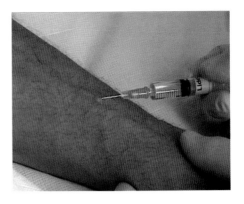

I Venous   II Arterial   III Central Venous   IV Airway   V Thoracic   VI Others   VII Supplemental Skills

I Venous   II Arterial   III Central Venous   IV Airway   V Thoracic   VI Others   VII Supplemental Skills

8. Subcutaneous Injection

Draw up the drugs first.

- Avoid administering drugs which you have not drawn up yourself – if you do have to then *always* check the contents and expiry date of the ampoule yourself.

Select a suitable injection site.

- Typical sites include skin of the: upper arm, abdomen, anterior thigh or buttock.
- When repeated subcutaneous injections are needed (e.g. insulin or heparin) use a hidden site to avoid unsightly bruises.
- Sites suitable for intradermal testing are similar to those for subcutaneous injections but also include the inner forearm and shoulder blades.

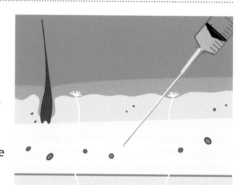

Prep the skin with an alcohol swab.

- Allowing the skin to dry before the injection is bactericidal as well as reducing the pain of injection.

Gently pinch the skin to elevate the subcutaneous fat.

- Raising a fold of skin by pinching with the non-dominant thumb and forefinger, will lift the adipose tissue away from the underlying muscle.

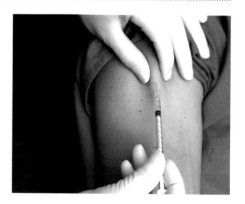

Insert the needle and inject the drug.

- Use a short (2 cm) 25- or 27 G needle, inserted at a 30° angle, through the epidermis.
- You may see a subcutaneous swelling, but the 'peau d'orange' (orange peel) appearance of intradermal injection should not be seen.
- Aspiration before injection is unnecessary before subcutaneous injection. Aspiration before administration of heparin increases the risk of local haematoma formation.

Remove the needle and observe for adverse reactions.

9. Venous Cutdown

Examine the leg for evidence of previous surgery to the veins.

- If the veins have been stripped, there may still be other collateral veins visible or palpable.
- Avoid using leg veins in a patient with significant pelvic or abdominal injury.

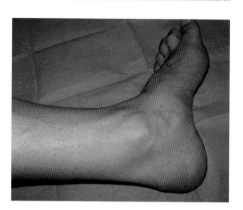

Prep the skin and infiltrate with local anaesthetic.

- The clinical situation may indicate that local anaesthesia is not required (e.g. if the patient is unconscious or time does not permit).

Palpate for the long saphenous vein 2 cm anterior and superior to the medial malleolus.

- You may not be able to see or feel the vein at all in an obese or shocked patient – however this is a reliable landmark.

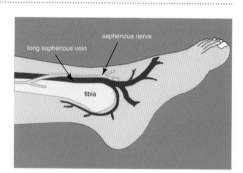

Make a 2 cm incision through the skin only, perpendicular to the direction of the vein, then expose and isolate the vein using blunt dissection with artery forceps.

- In a shocked patient the vein will be empty and may look and feel like the saphenous nerve which is immediately adjacent.

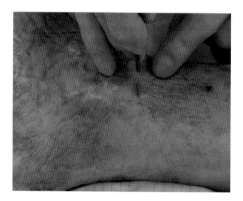

Pass the forceps under the vein and pull through two ligatures, then tie off the distal end of the vein as far distally as possible.

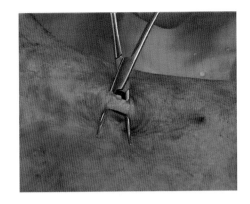

Now elevate the vein using the proximal ligature and incise it with a scalpel making a hole large enough to accommodate the intended cannula.

- Go carefully – you do not want to cut all the way through the vein.

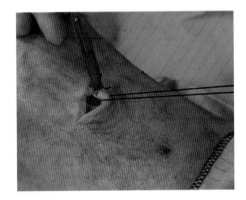

Using the largest cannula that will fit the vein, remove the needle, insert into the vein and secure with the tie.

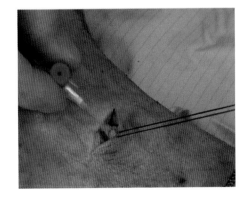

Connect the intravenous infusion and commence fluids.

- Set the rate of fluid infusion, it is likely to be very rapid at least initially, considering the clinical situation.

I Venous   II Arterial   III Central Venous   IV Airway   V Thoracic   VI Others   VII Supplemental Skills

Suture the wound either side of the cannula.

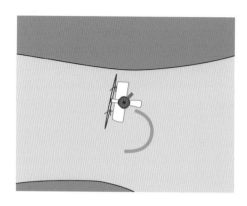

Apply a dressing. Have a large drink.

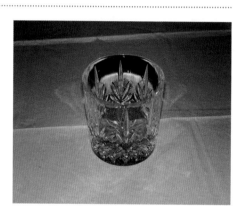

II
Arterial
Section

10. Arterial Blood Sampling

Position the hand comfortably with the wrist slightly extended, then palpate the radial artery carefully and prep the skin.

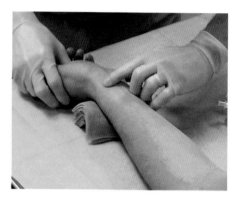

- The radial arterial pulse is most easily felt overlying the distal end of the radius. However, it may be palpated anywhere from the base of the thumb to the mid-forearm. Arterial blood gas (ABG) sampling can be successfully performed wherever a pulse can be palpated.

- Other possible sites for ABG sampling include: the femoral artery (groin); brachial artery (antecubital fossa); axillary artery (axilla); superficial temporal artery (temple); posterior tibial artery (ankle) or the dorsalis pedis artery (foot). Avoid the carotid artery as dislodgement of plaque within it could cause a stroke.

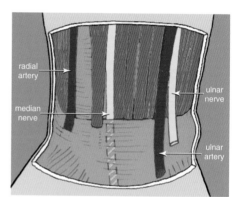

Now infiltrate with local anaesthetic over the intended puncture site.

- As well as being kind, local anaesthesia is important because pain could cause hyperventilation which can give spuriously low arterial CO_2 levels.
- If you puncture the artery with the local anaesthetic needle, it will make subsequent successful arterial puncture more difficult due to the haematoma.

Perform arterial puncture by advancing the needle at an angle of 45° to the skin towards the artery until blood flashes back into the syringe.

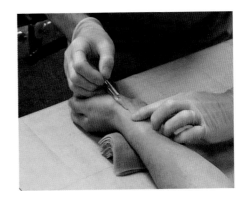

- Go slowly, the artery is more superficial than many people realise.
- If you have hit bone without getting blood back you may have transfixed the artery. All is not lost! The artery walls are thick and elastic. They do not collapse when a hole is made in the arterial wall. So withdraw the needle slowly and blood will appear when the needle tip re-enters the needle. For this reason, this 'transfixion technique' is just as effective as direct puncture, and is deliberately performed by some clinicians.

Steady the needle whilst the syringe fills with blood.

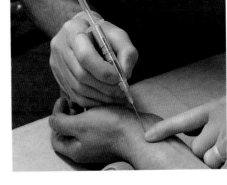

- Some ABG syringes are low-resistance, so blood under arterial pressure will fill the syringe without requiring aspiration.
- Other types of syringe seal at the plunger once blood reaches it – the plunger of this type of syringe should be drawn back a suitable volume (e.g. 2 ml prior to arterial puncture). The syringe then fills under arterial pressure and seals on contact with blood.
- If such a syringe is unavailable, take an ordinary 2 ml syringe, aspirate a small volume of 1:1000 heparin then empty the syringe which will leave enough heparin in the hub of the needle.

Withdraw the needle and immediately apply firm pressure for 5 min.

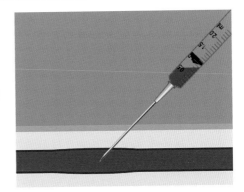

- Arterial pressure requires a well-formed platelet plug to prevent haemorrhage. This requires longer than the 2–3 min required to stop venous bleeding.

I Venous   II Arterial   III Central Venous   IV Airway   V Thoracic   VI Others   VII Supplemental Skills

11. Arterial Line Insertion

Gently extend the wrist and then feel for the arterial pulse.

- The arterial pulse is most easily felt overlying the radial head. However, it may be palpated anywhere from the base of the thumb to the mid-forearm. An arterial line can be successfully sited at any such place.

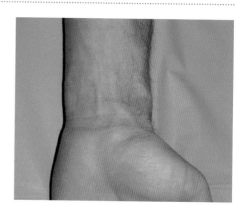

Prep the skin, then infiltrate the puncture site with local anaesthetic.

- The artery is very superficial. A common error is to go too deeply with local anaesthetic.
- If you puncture the artery with the local anaesthetic needle, it will make subsequent successful arterial cannulation more difficult because of haematoma formation.

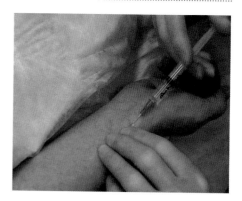

Piercing the skin with a needle eases the subsequent passage of the cannula.

- Again, take great care not to hit the artery with the needle.

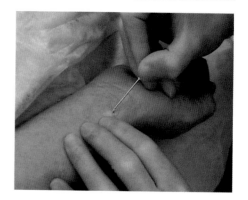

Whilst palpating the radial pulse insert the cannula towards the vessel. This should be done slowly at an acute angle – 20° or so to the skin.

- You may feel increased resistance as the needle enters the arterial wall, followed by much less resistance when the cannula is within the artery itself.

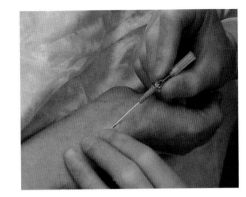

On entering the artery, withdraw the needle and advance the cannula into the vessel further along the artery.

- Try gently rotating the cannula as you advance it.

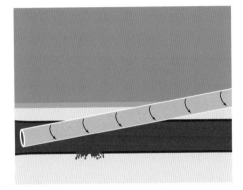

Compressing the artery at the cannula tip, remove the needle, then connect the arterial pressure tubing with a Luer lock device. Apply a dressing.

Aspirate to confirm arterial placement, remove any air bubbles and flush with saline.

- You must exclude all air bubbles from the line as inadvertent injection of air into an arterial line may cause distal ischaemia.

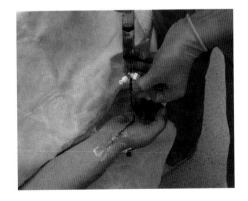

I Venous II Arterial III Central Venous IV Airway V Thoracic VI Others VII Supplemental Skills

I Venous   II Arterial   III Central Venous   IV Airway   V Thoracic   VI Others   VII Supplemental Skills

Secure the line with tape along the thumb.

- Pay great attention to all connections in this line – if a three-way tap is positioned incorrectly and the cap falls off, significant blood loss could occur.

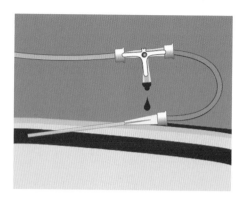

I Venous

II Arterial

III Central Venous

IV Airway

V Thoracic

VI Others

VII Supplemental Skills

III
Central Venous
Section

12. Internal Jugular Vein Cannulation

I Venous   II Arterial   III Central Venous   IV Airway   V Thoracic   VI Others   VII Supplemental Skills

Position the patient comfortably with head down tilt before prepping the skin and applying suitable drapes.

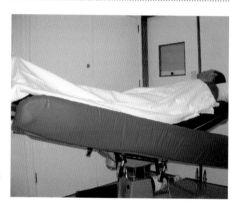

- If the patient is at risk of cardiac failure, then do not put them in the reverse Trendelenburg position. Instead, sit the patient up, then tip the whole bed head down. This has the overall effect of raising the patient's legs, which should elevate the Central Venous Pressure (CVP) without making a dyspnoeic patient feel worse.

- Alternatively delay head down tilt until just prior to needle insertion. Local anaesthesia and all preparations can be performed without head down tilt.

- Infection is an important complication of central venous cannulation which carries a significant morbidity (and even mortality). Use full aseptic precautions including gown, mask and gloves and do not be tempted to cut corners.

The point of insertion is mid-way between the insertion of the medial (sternal) head of sternocleidomastoid and the mastoid process behind the ear.

Infiltrate with local anaesthetic around the planned puncture site.

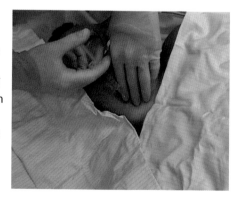

- You may find you locate the vein during this process.

- Some authorities recommend deliberate use of such a 'seeker' needle to locate the vein. This may reduce the chance of accidental carotid arterial puncture with a large (16G) needle.

- If there is any doubt, measure the blood pressure from this seeker needle – it should be $<20\,cmH_2O$.

Direct your needle in the sagittal plane, angled towards the feet, at an angle of about 45° from the vertical.

- The needle often passes through the most medial fibres of sternocleidomastoid.

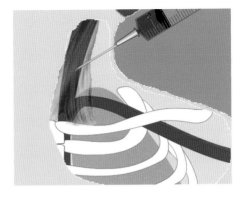

Align the introducer needle with your surface landmarks and advance towards the internal jugular vein whilst aspirating on the syringe.

- Placing a finger on the carotid artery and keeping your needle lateral to this will reduce the chance of arterial puncture.
- If you aspirate arterial blood, remove the needle and apply compression for at least 5 min to avoid causing a haematoma.

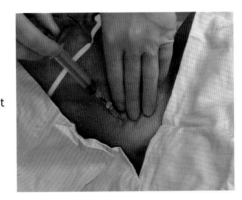

On entering the vein steady the needle and pass the guide wire through the syringe.

- If the patient is at risk of cardiac failure, at this point you can relieve the Trendelenburg positioning but take extra care to avoid air embolism during the subsequent line insertion.

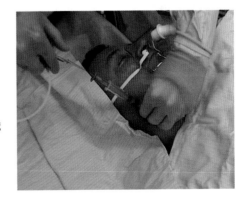

I Venous   II Arterial   III Central Venous   IV Airway   V Thoracic   VI Others   VII Supplemental Skills

Observe the ECG for cardiac arrhythmias provoked by the wire.

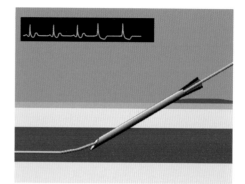

- Such arrhythmias are usually self-limiting. If this does occur, withdraw the wire until it stops.
- Very occasionally, the arrhythmia is more serious and prolonged. In this case treat as for the relevant arrhythmia.

Withdraw the syringe maintaining control of the wire at all times. Incise the skin immediately adjacent to the wire with a suitable scalpel blade. Pass the dilator over the wire and into the vein.

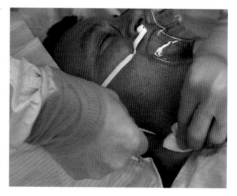

- Rotating the dilator as you pass it will usually make its passage smoother.

Remove the dilator before threading on the catheter and passing it down the wire.

- Keep hold of the wire at all times, you must be able to grab hold of the wire as it emerges from the end of the CVP catheter before you advance the catheter into the patient.
- If you lose the wire in the patient, you will need to go, cap in hand, to a radiologist who may retrieve it under X-ray control.

Position the catheter at an appropriate length for your patient (10-15 cm for adults). Withdraw the wire and immediately occlude and then cap the open lumen. Securely suture the line before applying a dressing.

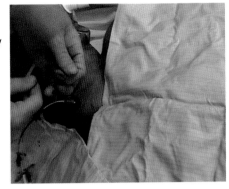

- If possible, suture the line in two separate points – this will reduce movement at the skin insertion point which in turn reduces the risk of infection.

Aspirate on all lumens to ensure that the air is removed and that there is free flow of venous blood, and then flush with saline.

I Venous   II Arterial   III Central Venous   IV Airway   V Thoracic   VI Others   VII Supplemental Skills

13. Low Approach to the Internal Jugular Vein

Position, prep and drape the patient as before.

Palpate and identify the two heads of sternocleidomastoid.

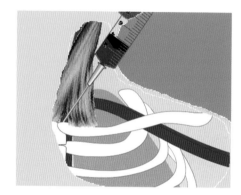

Infiltrate with local anaesthetic between the two heads, and then use a small 18G or 20G needle to locate the vessel. Advance the needle at right angles to the skin.

- You should find the vein less than 2 cm under the skin. Any deeper than this increases the risk of pneumothorax and is unnecessary.

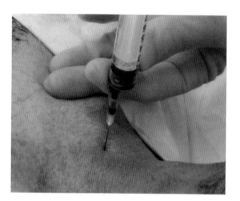

On locating the vein, detach the syringe from the needle.

- This provides a 'finder needle' which the larger introducer needle can go alongside.

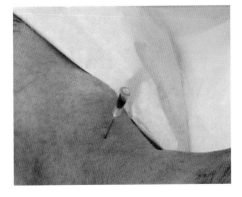

Now insert the introducer needle parallel to the finder needle.

Upon entering the vein, flatten the needle in line with the vessel and proceed with the standard Seldinger technique.

- Aspirate continuously as you flatten the needle to confirm that the tip of the needle is always in the vein. If you find you are suddenly unable to aspirate blood, stop, elevate the needle until you can once again aspirate, then try again.

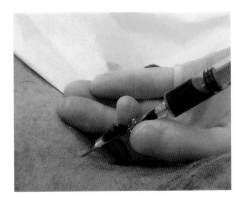

I Venous   II Arterial   **III Central Venous**   IV Airway   V Thoracic   VI Others   VII Supplemental Skills

14. Ultrasound-Guided Central Line

When using ultrasound guidance for internal jugular line placement position, prep and drape the patient in the usual way before infiltrating with local anaesthetic.

Roll up the sterile sheath for the ultrasound probe, then ask an assistant to drop gel onto the ultrasound probe before placing it in a sterile sheath.

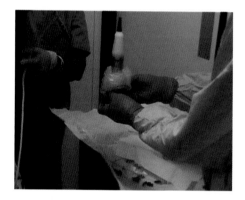

Secure the sheath, then apply gel to the probe from a sterile sachet.

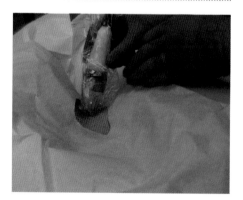

Scan the neck to identify the artery and vein. The vein will be seen to collapse easily under gentle pressure.

- Move the probe slowly and deliberately whilst applying moderate pressure.
- The artery is thicker walled, medial to the vein and pulsatile.

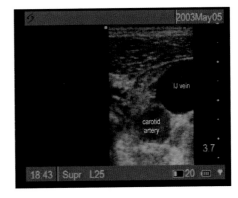

When the probe is aligned with the vein introduce the needle along the guide channel.

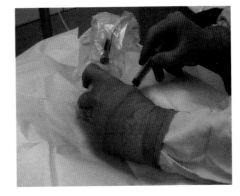

After entering the vein introduce the Seldinger wire as before.

- The wire may be viewed entering the vein on the ultrasound.

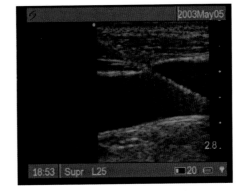

I Venous   II Arterial   **III Central Venous**   IV Airway   V Thoracic   VI Others   VII Supplemental Skills

15. Subclavian Vein Cannulation

Position the patient comfortably. Place a pack between the shoulder blades before positioning the arm and elevating the foot of the bed.

- If the patient is at risk of cardiac failure, then do not put them in the reverse Trendelenburg position. Instead, sit the patient up, then tip the whole bed head down. This has the overall effect of raising the patient's legs, which should elevate the Central Venous Pressure (CVP) without making a dyspnoeic patient feel worse.

- Alternatively only put the patient in the reverse Trendelenburg position for a brief period during the venous puncture until the wire is in place. Great care is then needed during catheter insertion and capping to avoid air embolism.

Prep the skin widely.

- Infection is an important complication of central venous cannulation which carries a significant morbidity (and even mortality). Use full aseptic precautions including gown, mask and gloves and do not be tempted to cut corners.

Check your landmarks before infiltrating with local anaesthetic.

- The insertion point for a subclavian central line is the junction of the medial 2/3 and lateral 1/3 of the clavicle. The needle should be directed medially and superiorly to pass under the clavicle into the vein. Aim for the tip of the opposite shoulder.

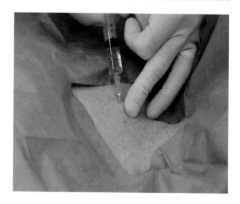

Take great care to avoid the underlying pleura. You may find the subclavian vein during this process but take care not to inject local anaesthetic directly into the vessel.

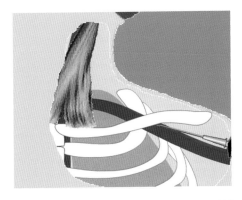

- The commonest serious complication of subclavian vein cannulation is pneumothorax. You *must* have a strategy to avoid this. Possibilities include:

  1. Placing a large sandbag between the patient's shoulder blades.

  2. Traction and external rotation of the ipsilateral arm.

  3. Applying a curve to the needle such that the tip of the introducer needle is always kept 'high'.

  4. Never directing the needle caudally – thus always aiming away from the apex of the lung (e.g. towards the contralateral shoulder tip).

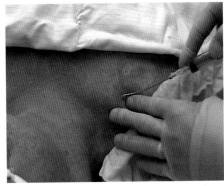

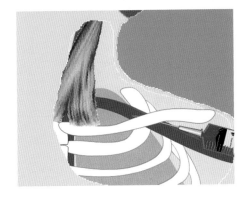

Advance the needle slowly towards the subclavian vein, aspirating gently on the syringe.

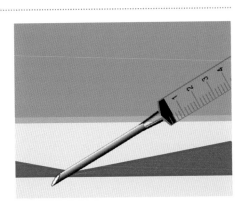

- The needle should be aimed at the sternal notch. Avoid angling the needle downward towards the apex of the lung.

- When a needle passes through a large (and therefore relatively thick-walled) vein, it may collapse the vein

I Venous   II Arterial   **III Central Venous**   IV Airway   V Thoracic   VI Others   VII Supplemental Skills

before transfixing both walls simultaneously – in which case no flashback of blood occurs. So go very slowly as you withdraw the needle, allowing the vein to refill so that you will aspirate blood if you have transfixed the vein. If, however, you withdraw too fast and 'miss' the vein a second time, you now have a large hole in both sides of the vein.

Pass the guidewire through the syringe. Observe the ECG for arrhythmias.

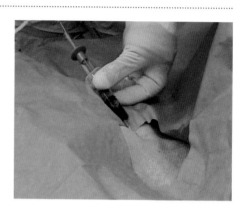

- Cardiac arrhythmias provoked by the wire are usually self-limiting – if you do provoke an arrhythmia, withdraw the wire until the arrhythmia stops.
- Very occasionally, the arrhythmia is not self-terminating. In this case treat as per standard protocols.

Withdraw the syringe whilst keeping control of the wire. Then incise the skin adjacent to the wire with a suitable scalpel. Advance the introducing dilator.

- Rotating the dilator as you pass it will usually make its passage smoother.
- A generous stab incision assists passage of the dilator but avoid lancing the vessel!

Now pass the catheter over the wire maintaining continuous control of the wire.

- Keep hold of the wire at all times, you must be able to grab hold of the wire as it emerges from the end before you advance the catheter into the patient.

Position the catheter at a suitable length for the patient.

- For an adult patient, rarely should more than 15 cm of catheter be inserted.

Withdraw the wire and immediately occlude and then cap the open lumen. Aspirate on each lumen before flushing with saline.

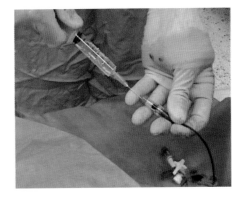

Finally, securely suture the line and apply a dressing.

- Suture the line in at least two separate points, this will reduce movement at the skin insertion point which, in turn, reduces the risk of infection.

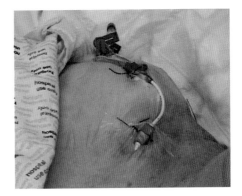

Obtain and review a CXR.

I Venous   II Arterial   III Central Venous   IV Airway   V Thoracic   VI Others   VII Supplemental Skills

16. Long Line Insertion

There are several options available to access the central circulation from a peripheral vein. These include a peripherally inserted central catheter (PICC line) and a Drum catheter.

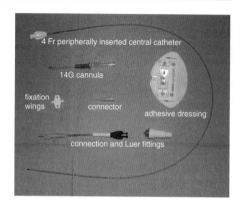

Insertion of a Drum catheter is described here. Apply a tourniquet and identify a suitable vein. The median basilic vein is best for long line insertion.

- It avoids potential obstruction as the catheter crosses the clavi-pectoral fascia.

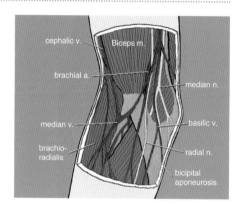

Prep the skin widely and position sterile drapes.

- Drapes have been left off in these photos for clarity of viewing.

I Venous   II Arterial   III Central Venous   IV Airway   V Thoracic   VI Others   VII Supplemental Skills

Infiltrate the skin with local anaesthetic.

- The major veins around the antecubital fossa are immediately subcutaneous, so a bleb of cutaneous local anaesthetic should be sufficient.

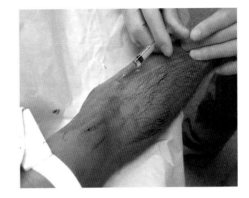

Cannulate the vein and aspirate blood to confirm correct position.

- Beware: the brachial artery lies very superficial, immediately deep to the bicipital aponeurosis.

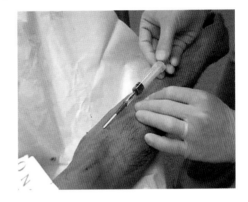

Advance the catheter over the needle into the vein. Get an assistant to release the tourniquet, then remove the needle whilst occluding the vein.

- This is a very large needle - be particularly careful to avoid sharp injury.

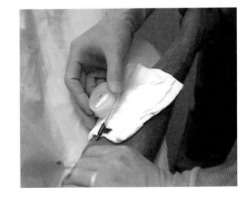

Insert the drum cartridge and advance the catheter, rotating the drum so that the curve of the catheter follows the vessel as it progresses medially.

- The clavi-pectoral fascia may limit proximal progress of the catheter. This is particularly likely if the catheter is in the cephalic rather than the basilic vein.
- To encourage the catheter to travel centrally, abduct and externally rotate the arm, then advance the catheter whilst applying pressure over the clavi-pectoral fascia.

I Venous   II Arterial   III Central Venous   IV Airway   V Thoracic   VI Others   VII Supplemental Skills

I Venous   II Arterial   III Central Venous   IV Airway   V Thoracic   VI Others   VII Supplemental Skills

- Get the patient to turn their head towards this side as you advance which should release tension in the clavi-pectoral fascia.

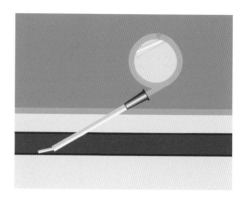

Observe the ECG for dysrhythmia suggesting the catheter has entered the right atrium.

Release the catheter drum and withdraw the cannula back over the catheter. Pressure may be needed at the puncture site to prevent bleeding. Withdraw the wire and immediately cap the catheter prior to aspirating all air and flushing with saline.

- The cannula of a long line contains several millilitre of air. Air embolism could be caused if the air is not carefully aspirated from the line prior to flushing.

Use the introducing wire laid superficially over the skin to approximate the position of the catheter tip in the superior venacava (SVC).

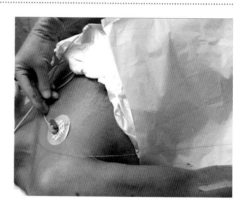

Obtain an X-ray to confirm the correct placement.

17. Femoral Vein Cannulation

The anatomical landmarks to facilitate reliable cannulation of the femoral vein are the inguinal ligament and the femoral artery.

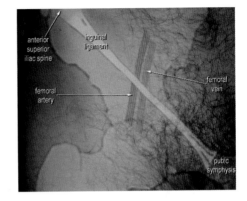

Position the patient comfortably with the leg slightly abducted. Prep the skin thoroughly and apply drapes.

- Use an alcoholic antiseptic solution and give it time to dry.
- Sterility is important here. Strict adherence to aseptic technique will increase the life of the line and reduce the patient's risk of sepsis. The groin is potentially 'dirtier' than the neck so ensure good sterile technique. Try to suture the line as far away from the groin as possible.
- Filling the veins prior to venous puncture is easier than with other central lines. You do not need head down tilt, but elevate the legs.

Palpate the femoral artery and infiltrate lidocaine just medial to it over the vein below the inguinal ligament.

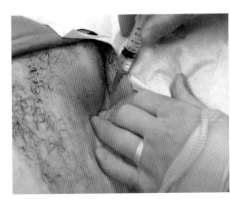

- You should always be able to feel a femoral artery pulse unless the patient is: profoundly hypotensive, morbidly obese or severely arteriopathic. The anatomy could be distorted in patients who have had previous groin surgery.
- If you cannot feel the femoral pulse consider using ultrasound guidance.
- Blind insertion *is* possible. The artery is at the midpoint between the anterior superior iliac spine and the pubic symphysis, so put a finger on that point and aim medial to that point.

Advance the needle towards the vein until free flow of venous blood is obtained.

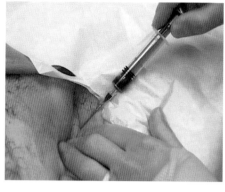

- On entering the vein if you do not get free and easy aspiration of blood you probably will not be able to advance the wire. Reposition the needle until aspiration is easy.
- If you accidentally puncture the artery, remove the needle and apply pressure for 5 min.
- If you cannot aspirate blood after your first pass, withdraw the needle very slowly whilst aspirating gently in case you have transfixed the vessel.

Introduce the wire then remove the needle.

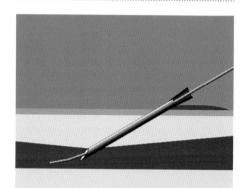

- ECG monitoring and the appearance of ectopic beats cannot be used during femoral line insertion to 'prove' the wire is located in a central vein as a 20 cm catheter will not reach the heart.

Incise the skin and railroad the dilator, then pass the catheter over the wire keeping control of the wire at all times.

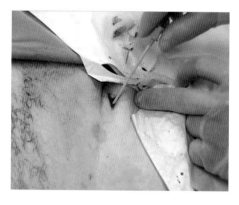

- The standard 20 cm line should be inserted to the hilt.
- A chest X-ray is not necessary as you should not be able to see the tip of the catheter on it. If you have good flow of venous blood under venous pressure that is sufficient to be able to use the line.

I Venous   II Arterial   III Central Venous   IV Airway   V Thoracic   VI Others   VII Supplemental Skills

Remove the wire and immediately occlude then cap the open lumen. Now aspirate and flush all lines.

- It is important to aspirate and flush every time drugs are injected into the catheter to confirm venous placement (lines can migrate through the vein wall or pull out).
- Aspiration also avoids the inadvertent administration of a drug bolus from the dead space of the line which is particularly important for patients receiving inotropes.
- Avoid mixing drugs in the same lumen. If this is unavoidable check compatibility first.

Suture the line in place.

- Suture the line in under aseptic conditions.
- Avoid the use of antibiotic ointments at the insertion site – they increase the rate of fungal colonisation and promote the development of antibiotic-resistant bacterial strains whilst having no effect on bloodstream infection rates.
- *However*, some units advocate the use of antifungal ointment over the puncture site of femoral dialysis lines.

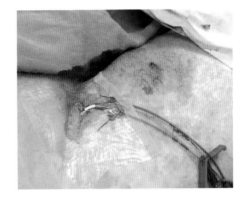

Apply a dressing:

- Use a sterile dressing to cover the wound.
- Remove the catheter when it is no longer required – on removal send the catheter tip for culture.
- Femoral lines may increase the risk of deep venous thrombosis so remove them as soon as possible.

I Venous   II Arterial   III Central Venous   IV Airway   V Thoracic   VI Others   VII Supplemental Skills

IV
Airway
Section

18. Basic Airway Management

I Venous

II Arterial

III Central Venous

IV Airway

V Thoracic

VI Others

VII Supplemental Skills

If your patient is either apnoeic or obstructed you need to establish a clear, open airway.

- Clear the airway first – look inside the mouth and remove any obvious foreign bodies.

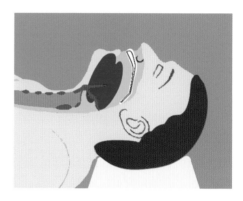

- Use suction – turn on the suction (even if it is not required right now) and place the Yankauer sucker under the patient's pillow. You must ensure that the patient does not regurgitate or vomit during your airway interventions as aspiration of stomach contents may cause potentially fatal aspiration pneumonitis.

- Get some assistance and apply basic monitoring to the patient.

Give oxygen at 10 l/min continuously.

- Use the piped wall supply if available – an oxygen cylinder will run out quite quickly at 10 l/min.

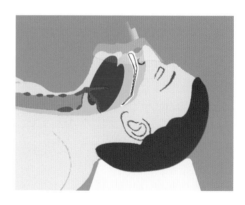

- Use an oxygen mask with a rebreathing bag if one is available (see equipment) as you will be able to give higher concentrations of oxygen than with standard oxygen masks.

First, lift the chin, then perform a jaw thrust by placing fingers behind the mandible and displacing it anteriorly.

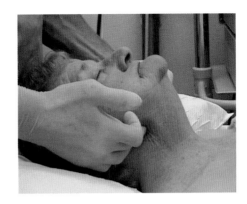

- It is usually easier to open the mouth, then perform jaw thrust, then close the mouth with the lower incisors (if present) now in front of the upper incisors.
- In some patients (particularly the obese), performing chin lift and/or jaw thrust may require considerable force which may be poorly tolerated by awake or semi-conscious patients.

Next correctly size and introduce a Guedel airway.

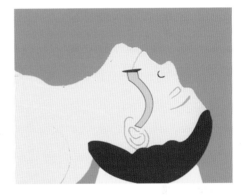

- The oropharyngeal airway is measured from the edge of the mouth to the tragus. Too small an airway will not get past the tongue. Too large an airway may become obstructed up against the anterior pharyngeal wall.
- To get the oropharyngeal airway past the tongue, insert it upside-down, then rotate into the correct position once past the tongue.

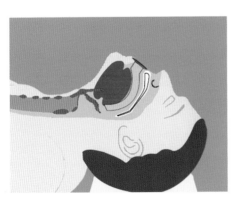

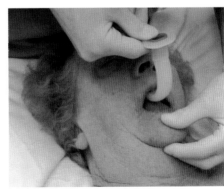

I Venous   II Arterial   III Central Venous   IV Airway   V Thoracic   VI Others   VII Supplemental Skills

If the airway remains obstructed, try a nasopharyngeal airway which should be aimed posteriorly with gentle sustained pressure parallel to the floor of the nasal cavity.

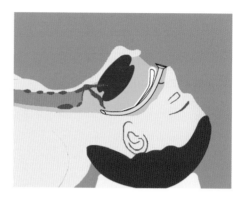

- To start with, use a 6 mm airway for females and a 7 mm airway for males.
- Try to identify which the most patent nostril is and start with that side.

Apply gel, and then introduce the airway into the nares. Aiming directly posteriorly, apply continuous but gentle pressure into the nostril to help get the nasopharyngeal airway past the turbinates.

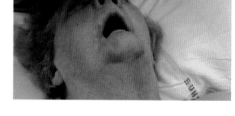

- Do not apply undue force, you will only cause epistaxis.
- You may feel the resistance suddenly 'giving way' as the airway emerges into the oropharynx.
- If your brand of nasopharyngeal airway does not have large enough flanges, insert a safety pin through the flanges to prevent it being pushed right into the nares.

Apply a mask and either confirm unobstructed spontaneous ventilation or ventilate using a close-fitting face mask and an Ambubag if necessary.

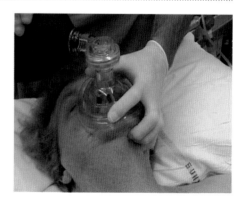

- Getting a good 'seal' around the close-fitting face mask may be impossible in bearded patients – try applying a large adhesive dressing (e.g. Opsite®) over the beard, then cut a hole for the nose and mouth and reapply the mask.

- For edentulous patients, use a Guedel airway, but also consider leaving the dentures in if they are close-fitting.

I Venous   II Arterial   III Central Venous   IV Airway   V Thoracic   VI Others   VII Supplemental Skills

If these simple techniques for airway control fail, you must proceed to more advanced airway management.

- Call an anaesthetist but prepare to intubate the patient yourself if none is available.

19. Endotracheal Intubation

Think why you are intubating this patient: Is it to allow ventilation of the lungs (head injury, apnoea); or to protect their lungs from blood (blood in the airway) or gastric contents (decreased level of consciousness)?

- Consider the use of cricoid pressure (Sellick's manoeuvre). This is downward pressure by your assistant, on the cricoid cartilage until the tube is confirmed as being in the trachea.

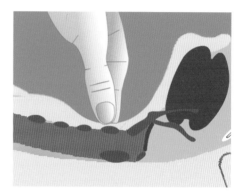

- The aim of cricoid pressure is to compress the oesophagus between the cricoid ring, which is the only complete cartilaginous ring in the airway, and the sixth cervical vertebral body, thereby preventing reflux of stomach contents into the larynx.

- Avoid using cricoid pressure if the patient is actively vomiting, as this could cause oesophageal rupture.

Do you need to give drugs to facilitate intubation?

- A semi-conscious patient may not allow you to put a laryngoscope or endotracheal tube (ETT) in their mouth – if they need to be sedated and paralyzed, you should call upon a friendly anaesthetist who will help you out.

- Alternatively, a nasotracheal tube could be passed down one nostril but this is an advanced airway skill requiring considerable practice. It should never be performed for the first time on a critically ill patient who needs their airway controlling emergently.

Check you have a functional laryngoscope, a range of sizes of ETT and medical suction which works.

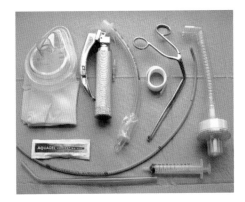

- *Always* check all your equipment before use. Laryngoscope bulbs can be blown, ETT cuffs can be perforated and suction apparatus may be disconnected. All of these may cause delay, which puts the patient at increased risk of hypoxia.

Position the patient with a pillow behind the neck.

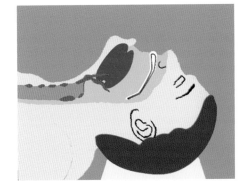

- The 'sniffing the morning air' position aligns the airway into as straight a line as possible. Think of the neck as having just two joints, one at the bottom with the thorax – which should be flexed, and one at the top with the head – which should be extended. A pillow can do this most effectively. However, more than one pillow may be too much.
- *Caution*! Avoid neck movement in patients with real or potential injury to the cervical spine.
- Turn the sucker on and place it under the pillow – it can do no harm yet could save vital seconds aspirating stomach contents or blood from the oropharynx.

Consider pre-oxygenating the patient.

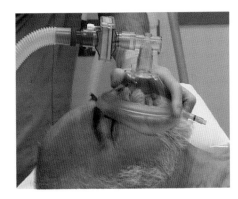

- During intubation, the patient is apnoeic and certainly at risk of hypoxia. Therefore give yourself the biggest safety margin by pre-oxygenating the patient with 100% oxygen given via a 'bag-valve-mask' device such as an Ambubag® for 3 min. This may 'buy' you as much as 3 min. extra oxygenation during apnoea mostly because of the increase in oxygen content of the lungs (do the maths – 3 l of air contains $3 \times 21\% = 0.65\,l$ oxygen compared with 3 l oxygen).

I Venous   II Arterial   III Central Venous   IV Airway   V Thoracic   VI Others   VII Supplemental Skills

- Full pre-oxygenation is only achieved with a tight-fitting mask and seal, otherwise atmospheric air is entrained and dilutes the oxygen.

With the laryngoscope in your left hand extend the head with your right so that the mouth falls open. Then insert the laryngoscope into the right side of the mouth, bring it into the midline and advance it.

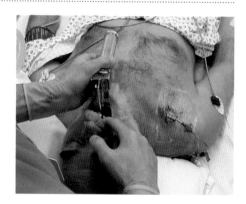

- This manoeuvre moves the tongue to the left of the mouth out of your field of vision.

Locate the epiglottis, then position the tip of the laryngoscope anterior to the epiglottis.

- Hold your breath when you start to intubate. When you need to take a breath, so does the patient! Stop your attempts and revert to oxygenation with a bag and mask.

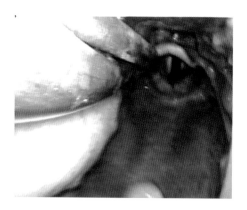

Check that you have not trapped the lips with your blade.

- You can cause a significant laceration of the lips with the steel laryngoscope blade.

Now push your arm away from you to expose the vocal cords. *Do not lever the scope on the teeth*.

- Tremendous pressure can be bought to bear on the incisors in this way. Patients do not like having their teeth damaged during their hospital admission. It often leads to litigation.

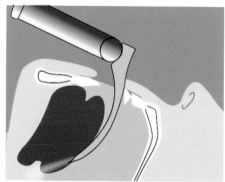

Insert the ETT between the vocal cords until the cuff is just passed the cords.

- In adult males, an 8.0-mm internal diameter ETT is appropriate, while in adult females a 7.0-mm ETT is generally suitable.

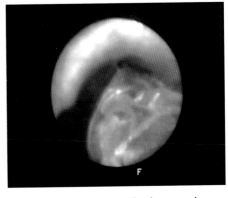

- If you can see the laryngeal inlet but cannot pass a tube because the laryngoscope is obscuring the view or because teeth are in the way, intubate the trachea with a bougie and then slide the ETT over the bougie into the trachea. In time you may become skilled with a bougie and can then use it to intubate the trachea when you cannot see the laryngeal inlet at all.

Remove the scope carefully.

- The teeth and lips can be damaged on the way out as well as on the way in.

Connect your breathing system and inflate the lungs with 100% oxygen.

- Formulate a backup plan every time you intubate a patient for the possibility that endotracheal intubation may fail. Depending on your experience, this could be an insertion of a laryngeal mask airway; cricothyroidotomy; or, if you are desperate, a surgeon may need to perform emergency tracheostomy. *Do not* persist with unsuccessful attempts. If you cannot intubate the trachea after two attempts, continue bag and mask ventilation with 100% oxygen and call for more experienced help.

Ask your assistant to inflate the cuff until an air leak around the tube is no longer audible.

- Do not over-inflate the cuff as this can cause pressure necrosis of the tracheal mucosa.

Check that the tube is at an appropriate distance and that both lungs are inflating.

- For adult males, the tube should inserted until the 24-cm mark is at the teeth, for females 22 cm. However, this is approximate. Listen to both sides of the chest to confirm that the tube is in the trachea but has not gone past the carina. If there is any doubt, a chest X ray will confirm the position of the ETT tip.
- Uncuffed ETT tubes are generally used in children under 8 years of age. ETT size in children may be estimated using the formula $x = age/4 + 4$. ETT length at the teeth is $y = age/2 + 12$ estimated by $age/2 + 12$.

I Venous   II Arterial   III Central Venous   IV Airway   V Thoracic   VI Others   VII Supplemental Skills

I Venous   II Arterial   III Central Venous   **IV Airway**   V Thoracic   VI Others   VII Supplemental Skills

Perform confirmatory tests including auscultation over the lungs and stomach and identifying expired CO_2.

- When you are sure the tube is in the right place, you need to consider the patient's future management. Are they breathing spontaneously, or more likely, do they need ventilating? Any intubated patient certainly needs to be managed in a critical care area, so contact the intensive care team for further advice.

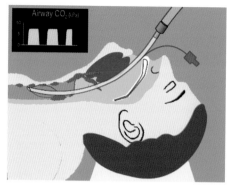

Secure the tube with tape or a tie.

- You only have to have one tube fall out before you become much better at securing them!

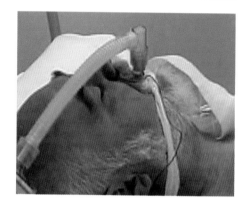

20. Laryngeal Mask Airway Insertion

Ensure adequate pre-oxygenation using a mask and AMBUbag connected to an oxygen supply.

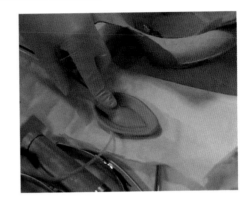

- Three minutes pre-oxygenation will usually ensure the oxygen content of the lungs is >90%, but if time is short, four vital capacity breaths are also effective if you have an air-tight seal.

- Check the laryngeal mask airway before use – inflate the cuff and discard if there is a leak.

- Check the tubing and cuff of a reusable LMA for signs of perishing caused by repeated autoclaving.

- Always have medical suction immediately available.

Prepare the mask by deflating the cuff and applying a small amount of water-based lubricant.

- The lubricant should be primarily applied to the posterior surface of the LMA which will pass over the posterior pharyngeal wall.

- The reusable LMA is autoclaved between uses. A maximum of 40 uses is recommended (i.e. 39 re-uses). A record should be kept of how often the LMA has been used – this requires identification of individual LMAs.

- There are disposable LMAs available but they do not all have identical characteristics to the classic LMA.

Extend the head slightly to open the mouth. This may be aided if necessary.

- This can effectively be done by pushing on the occiput with one hand whilst inserting the LMA with the other.

I Venous   II Arterial   III Central Venous   IV Airway   V Thoracic   VI Others   VII Supplemental Skills

Hold the mask like a pen in gloved hands with the index finger extended to the junction of cuff and tube.

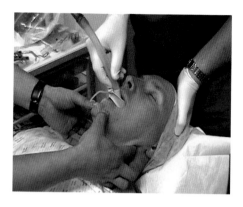

- Always wear gloves during airway management.

Insert the LMA maintaining pressure with the index finger. A slight twist may aid passage past the soft palate.

- Good lubrication is important here.
- Be careful not to catch the upper lip as you push the LMA in – it is easy to lacerate the lip.

Inflate the cuff slowly with the correct volume of air. Correct placement is suggested with a slight outward movement of the mask.

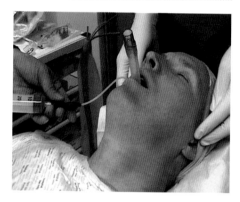

- Different size masks and manufacturers require different volumes of air so check the instructions.
- Cricoid pressure may prevent correct positioning – so if using an LMA during resuscitation, release cricoid pressure if the airway is not patent following insertion and inflation.

After confirming successful pulmonary ventilation secure the mask with tape.

- Keep the mask inflated until it is removed.
- Remove the LMA only when the patient is conscious with intact airway reflexes.

If lung ventilation is inadequate, the most likely cause is poor positioning of the cuff within the larynx. The epiglottis can be folded down by the LMA to obstruct the laryngeal inlet.

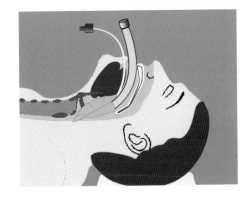

Try the following remedial measures:

- Deflate then re-inflate the cuff.
- Remove the mask, suction the oropharynx, then re-insert.
- Try a different size LMA – usually larger but sometimes smaller.

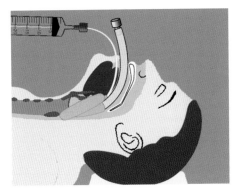

I Venous II Arterial III Central Venous IV Airway V Thoracic VI Others VII Supplemental Skills

21. Cricothyroidotomy

If a patient requires oxygenation and you cannot achieve this by simple means (face mask, Ambubag®, oropharyngeal or nasopharyngeal airways) or by more invasive means (endotracheal intubation, laryngeal mask airway insertion), they need a surgical airway.

- A patient should *never* die of an obstructed airway without an attempt being made to create a surgical airway.
- The options available are: formal tracheostomy, surgical cricothyroidotomy or needle cricothyroidotomy, depending on the time and experience available.
- Cricothyroidotomy is the easiest of the surgical airways to create because only subcutaneous fat lies between the skin and the cricothyroid membrane.
- Needle cricothyroidotomy is used as a last resort to buy time whilst a more formal surgical airway can be created.

This is a life-threatening emergency. The patient will be cyanosed.

- There is a significant chance that the patient will not survive. Do not think you will always succeed on your own. Send someone to get a surgeon capable of formal tracheostomy. However, do not wait for them – the patient could have died by the time they arrive.
- A cricothyroidotomy should be achievable in less than a minute even in the emergency situation when a patient is tachypnoeic and even combative due to hypoxia (they get progressively less combative as they become more hypoxic).
- Wear gown/gloves/eye protection as appropriate.

Extend the head and place a sandbag under the patient's shoulders unless the patient has a neck injury.

- Head extension will improve your operating position considerably.
- You may only have time to remove the pillow from under the patient's head.

Palpate the thyroid and cricoid cartilages.

- It is crucial that you can feel these landmarks. You must know you are in the midline and at the right level in order to identify the cricothyroid membrane.

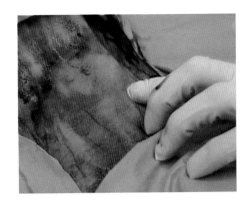

Make a 1-cm transverse incision straight through into the trachea.

- You may not have time or need for local anaesthesia here as the patient may not be conscious. However, if there is time and if the patient is conscious, infiltrate local anaesthetic in the midline.

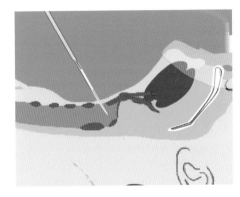

Use the scalpel handle to dilate the hole.

- Rotate the handle gently within the hole in the trachea.

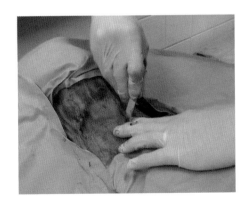

Now introduce the tube – check for exhaled CO_2 and once you have confirmed the tube is in the trachea, ventilate with 100% oxygen. Secure the tube so that it cannot fall out.

- Colorimetric CO_2 detector devices are available which detect CO_2 by using a pH sensitive indicator if you do not have access to a capnograph. These have been validated for use in the Emergency Room.

- In the absence of a CO_2 detector, use clinical signs to confirm tracheal placement: chest expansion, 'fogging' of the tube on expiration and bilateral breath sounds.

In a dire emergency, you can perform needle cricothyroidotomy. This can 'buy' you 30 or so minutes whilst you secure a definitive surgical airway.

- There are various methods of achieving this – at its simplest it involves using a 14G IV cannula, a three-way tap and a length of oxygen tubing.

- Another variation is to use the barrel of a 2 ml syringe which is inserted into the Luer fitting of the 14G cannula. Oxygen tubing with a small side-hole cut a few inches from the end is wedged into the syringe barrel.

- Proprietary kits are available for performing needle cricothyroidotomy.

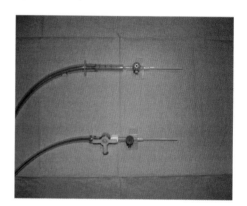

Introduce a 14G cannula, connected to a 10 ml syringe containing saline, through the cricothyroid membrane.

- Aspirate after skin penetration – when air is aspirated, remove the needle and syringe – then advance the cannula into the trachea.

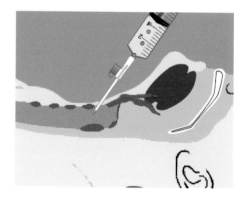

Connect a three-way tap and fit standard green oxygen tubing over the Luer fitting of the three-way tap.

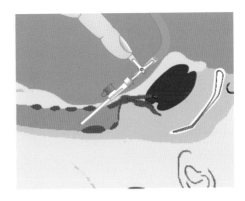

- Ensure you retain absolute control of the cannula – it must not fall out at this stage.

Turn on the oxygen at 10 l/min. Occlude the open lumen of the three-way tap for 1 s, then off for 4 s.

Call for help to secure a more definitive airway.

Now book a holiday to the Caribbean.

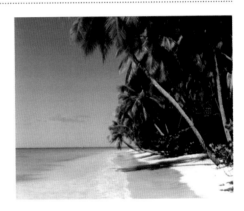

I Venous   II Arterial   III Central Venous   IV Airway   V Thoracic   VI Others   VII Supplemental Skills

V
Thoracic Section

I Venous

II Arterial

III Central Venous

IV Airway

V Thoracic

VI Others

VII Supplemental Skills

22. Chest Drain Insertion

Position the patient either sitting forward or semi-recumbent.

- Patient positioning is important. The common positions are sitting with the arms forward or lying semi-recumbent with the arm behind the head.

- There is a 'safe triangle' for insertion bordered by the anterior border of latissimus dorsi, the lateral border of pectoralis major and the level of the nipple.

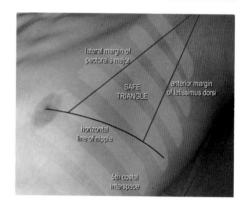

- The mid-axillary line within this triangle is the optimal site for insertion.

Use strict aseptic technique:

- Administer appropriate antibiotics if indicated (e.g. for traumatic haemothorax drainage).
- Check the patient's coagulation status before you start unless this is an emergency.

Infiltrate the skin and subcutaneous tissues with local anaesthetic. Go down onto the lower rib with your local anaesthetic.

- This procedure is very painful without proper pain relief. Use local anaesthesia generously, give it time to work properly and consider the use of sedatives or analgesics if appropriate.

- Patients with chronic obstructive pulmonary disease are particularly at risk of respiratory depression with sedative drugs.

- It does not matter if you aspirate pleural fluid with the local anaesthetic.

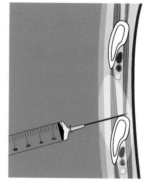
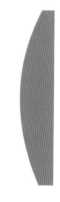
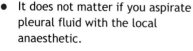

- Do not be surprised if the patient coughs during this process.

Incise the chest wall 2 cm below the proposed site of insertion.

- Make your incision appropriate for the size of chest tube you are inserting.
- If you are putting in a small drain, you should not insert a gloved finger into the thorax (as the incision would need to be much larger for this). Instead perform blunt dissection using forceps all the way into the thorax.
- Use a size 24Fr gauge chest drain or greater to drain a haemothorax as this allows on-going assessment of blood loss and is less likely to become blocked by blood clot. A 14-18Fr drain is perfectly adequate for pneumothorax drainage.

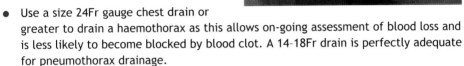

Perform blunt dissection using artery forceps through into the pleural cavity.

For a large (>24Fr) chest drain, sweep the tip of the index finger around to ensure the lung is not adherent to the insertion site.

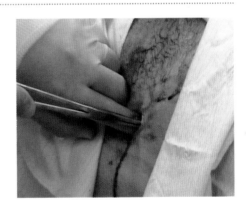

Remove and discard the trocar from the drain.

- Some chest drains come with a flexible trocar, thus reducing the risk of lung trauma.

Insert the drain into the pleural cavity and slide into position.

- Aim for the apex if you are treating pneumothorax, whereas the basal region is more suitable if draining fluid.

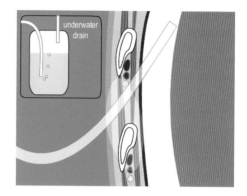

Connect the drain to an underwater seal device.

- If no underwater seal is available, or during transport of the patient, use a one-way (Heimlich) valve.
- The bottles of the underwater seal must always be below the level of the chest – otherwise the contents of the drain bottle will be siphoned into the chest.
- Avoid clamping the chest drain when moving or transporting a patient. You can cause a significant pneumothorax to re-accumulate especially if people forget to remove the clamp after the patient has been moved.

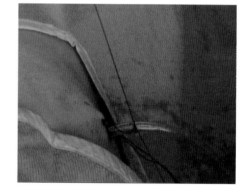

- Be suspicious if the fluid in the chest drain tubes has stopped 'swinging' with respiration. The absence of oscillations may indicate obstruction of the drainage system by clots or kinks, loss of sub-atmospheric pressure or complete re-expansion of the lung.
- Always take extra care with a patient with a chest drain who is being ventilated. It is very easy to convert a simple pneumothorax to a tension pneumothorax with positive pressure ventilation.

Suture the drain in position and apply a dressing.

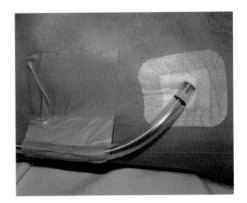

- 'Purse string' sutures are not recommended any more – close the wound with one or two skin sutures and apply a dressing. An 'omental tag' fixation technique supports the tube whilst allowing it to lie a little way from the chest wall.

- Get a chest X-ray after chest tube insertion to assess the chest tube position and whether or not it has successfully treated the problem.

23. Pleural Tap

Make the diagnosis clinically – or radiologically with X-ray or ultrasound. A lateral decubitus X-ray film will indicate how much fluid there is.

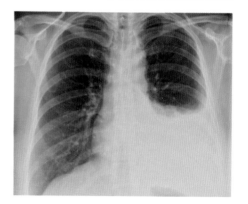

- If there is only a small amount of fluid, but it needs draining for diagnostic or therapeutic reasons, then it may be better to use ultrasound to ascertain where the effusion is maximal (see Pleural fluid drainage animation).

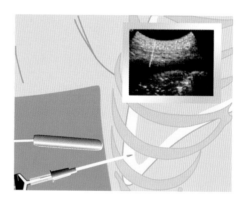

Check that you have all the required equipment, that you are familiar with its use and that it is correctly assembled.

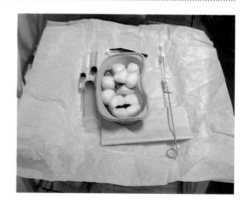

- Different manufacturers have different instructions for use so read these carefully.

Prep the skin widely around the 5th intercostal space in the mid-axillary line.

- Thoracentesis is best performed with the patient sitting comfortably, leaning slightly forward and resting the arms on a support. Performing it with the patient lying down is possible but more difficult, possibly requiring ultrasound or CT guidance.

Percuss the chest to confirm the stony dullness of a pleural effusion.

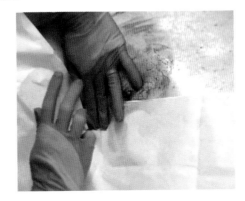

Infiltrate the skin and subcutaneous tissues with lidocaine using a fine gauge needle. Now infiltrate more deeply with an 18 G needle – aim to strike the rib. Inject more lidocaine and walk off the rib superiorly to avoid the intercostals vessels and nerves of the rib above.

- Use plenty of local anaesthetic – this includes the periosteum of the rib and the parietal pleura which are both sensitive structures. As the lung expands against the chest wall, the patient may feel pleuritic pain.
- You may aspirate pleural fluid during this process.

Now aspirate fluid for diagnostics and transfer to appropriate bottles for biochemistry, cytology and microbiology.

- If this is a diagnostic procedure, a 20 ml syringe and green 21 G needle may be sufficient. However, if this is therapeutic, then a proprietary set such as this may be used. A 50 ml syringe, three-way tap and plastic cannula are perfectly adequate if you only intend aspirating fluid.
- When removing the needle, ask the patient to perform a Valsalva manoeuvre to reduce the possibility of pneumothorax developing.

- Analysis of the fluid should make the diagnosis of exudate or transudate. A transudate is defined as total protein pleural fluid-serum ratio of 0.5, Lactate dehydrogenase (LDH) pleural fluid-serum ratio <0.6, absolute pleural fluid LDH <200 IU or <2/3 of the normal serum level.

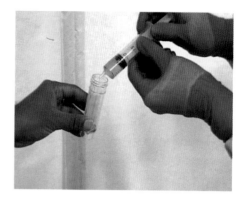

If you are just doing a diagnostic tap simply apply a plaster over the puncture site. If proceeding to formal drainage proceed to incise the skin with a scalpel blade. Now introduce the catheter over the trocar introducer striking the rib and then entering the pleural cavity over its superior border.

- Entering the pleural cavity above the rib avoids causing damage to the intercostal vessels and nerve.

Once in the pleural cavity withdraw the trocar before advancing the catheter over the introducer stylet. Suture the catheter securely in place. Then connect a three-way tap with a 50 ml syringe and sterile tubing leading to a suitable collection vessel.

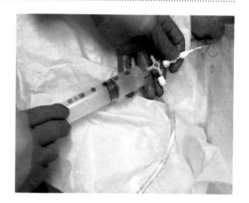

Aspirate fluid up to a maximum of 1500 ml at any one time.

- Stop the procedure if severe pain, breathlessness, bradycardia, faintness or other significant symptoms occur, even if a substantial amount of fluid remains in the chest.
- Withdrawing more than 1500 ml of pleural fluid all at one go has been associated with the development of pulmonary oedema.

Apply a dressing:

Obtain chest X-rays after thoracentesis in order to: document fluid removal; view the lung parenchyma previously obscured by the fluid and to search for possible complications of the procedure.

- X-rays taken in expiration are more likely to reveal a small pneumothorax.

24. Needle Thoracentesis

Suspect a tension pneumothorax with any of the following:

- Appropriate history:
  - Penetrating chest wounds.
  - Post-surgical (renal, thoracic or diaphragmatic).
  - Status asthmaticus.
  - Chronic obstructive pulmonary disease (COPD).

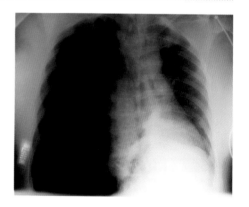

- Symptoms and signs:
  - Worsening hypoxia and tachypnoea.
  - Tracheal deviation to the opposite side.
  - Poor expansion of both sides, but especially the ipsilateral side.
  - Absent breath sounds ipsilaterally.
  - Hyper-resonant to percussion ipsilaterally.
  - Unexplained hypotension.
  - Distended neck veins.

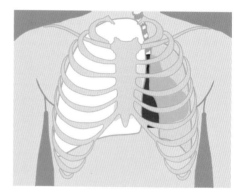

If immediately available, administer oxygen 12 l/min using a non-rebreathing mask or positive pressure with bag-valve-mask.

- However, do not waste time waiting for oxygen or other equipment. This is a life-threatening condition which demands immediate intervention.
- This is the emergency treatment for tension pneumothorax. It should be followed by insertion of a formal chest drain.
- The diagnosis should never need to be made radiologically. It must always be considered when a patient has this history and these clinical signs.

Identify the 2nd intercostal space, and the mid-clavicular line. The 1st rib cannot normally be felt. The 2nd rib is felt just below the collar bone.

- It is not absolutely crucial which interspace the needle passes through.

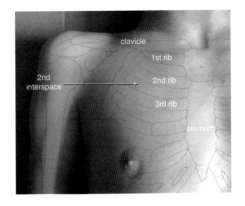

Insert the needle just over the 3rd rib, through the intercostal muscles and into the chest cavity.

- An Angiocath-type (catheter-over-cannula) needle is normally used, mounted on a syringe.
- A 'hiss' of air confirms the diagnosis of tension pneumothorax and this decompression should give immediate relief.

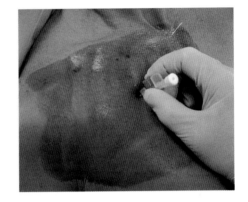

Slide the catheter over the needle and into the chest cavity. Attach a syringe and aspirate all the free air.

- Aspirate as much air as necessary to relieve the patient's acute symptoms.
- Leave the catheter in place so you can remove more free air as it accumulates until a formal drain is in place.

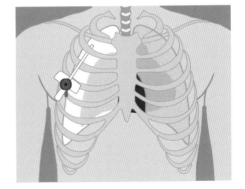

- If a formal chest drain is not available a Heimlich valve can be used. This is a flap valve which allows air to pass out of the chest but prevents air entry.

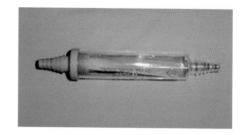

Now go and change your underwear.

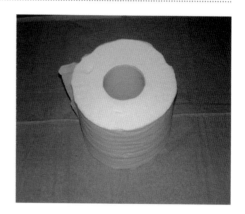

25. Spirometry

Apply a nasal clip to the subject's nose.

- Forced vital capacity and vital capacity values vary with the position of the patient. These variables can be 7–8 % greater in patients who are sitting during the test compared with patients who are supine. Forced vital capacity is about 2% greater in patients who are standing compared with patients who are supine.

Ensure that the spirometer is switched on and loaded with paper. Fit a new clean mouthpiece.

- To determine the validity of spirometric results, at least three acceptable spirograms must be obtained, but do them on the same paper. Ignore and repeat obvious outliers.

- To avoid cross-contamination, reusable mouthpieces, breathing tubes, valves and manifolds should be disinfected or sterilised regularly.

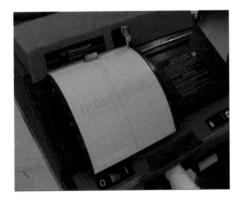

Instruct the subject to take a maximal breath in and then blow out as fast and for as long as they can.

- Considerable patient effort and cooperation is required to get meaningful results. So you must be enthusiastic throughout the test, reinforcing and encouraging the patient through their attempts at spirometry.

- Beware the patient who 'coughs' or 'pea shoots' into the mouthpiece.

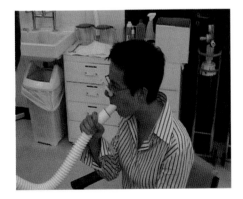

Repeat for three good quality recordings on the same paper.

- Once the patient has completed three spirograms, label the chart with the patient's name and the date.

- Take the average of three good quality recordings.

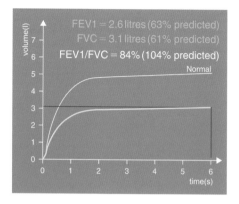

VI
Others
Section

I Venous

II Arterial

III Central Venous

IV Airway

V Thoracic

VI Others

VII Supplemental Skills

26. Lumbar Puncture

Position the patient comfortably on their side, the head should be flexed and their knees drawn up to their chest.

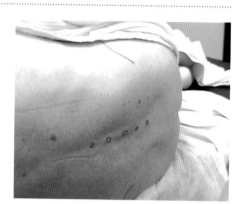

- You can try asking them to curl up 'like an angry cat' or to 'put their knees up to their chest and chin right down on their chest'.
- Get an assistant to help to encourage the patient to do this and maintain their position.
- Careful positioning is the key to success with lumbar puncture.

Choose the type and diameter of your spinal needle carefully.

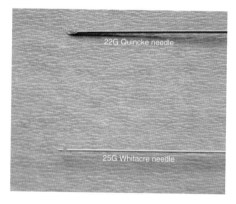

22G Quincke needle

25G Whitacre needle

- Needles with a non-cutting tip or pencil point (Whitacre or Sprotte) which part the dural fibres rather than cut them are associated with a lower incidence of post-dural puncture headache.
- The smaller the diameter of the needle, the lower the leakage of cerebrospinal fluid (CSF) and therefore the lower the risk of the patient developing a post-lumbar puncture headache.
- However, the needle lumen has to be large enough to allow potentially thick fluid such as pus in meningitis to flow and to allow accurate measurement of pressure. If you suspect meningitis a 20G needle is best.
- A 22G pencil-point needle is appropriate for most diagnostic taps.

Palpate the level of the fourth lumbar vertebra in the line of the iliac crest (Tuffier's line).

- This is not absolute but a reasonable guide to the L3/4 interspace.
- The spinal cord ends at L1-2 so take care to stay below this level.
- Look for evidence of spina bifida occulta (e.g. sacral cleft or hairy skin patch) over the lumbar spine. This is associated with a low-tethered spinal cord.

Prep the skin.

- Chlorhexidine in alcohol is a more effective antiseptic than iodine.
- The alcoholic chlorhexidine must dry in order to be effective.
- It is imperative that excess alcohol is not tracked by the needle to the subarachnoid space.

Apply the sterile drape.

- Ensure the local anaesthetic solution, needles and bottles are ready before you start.

Confirm the landmarks before infiltrating with local anaesthetic between the two spinous processes.

- You may find it easier to identify the interspace using two fingers – one either side of the space – rather than one finger in the space.

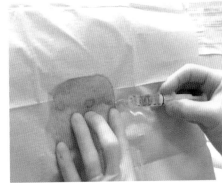

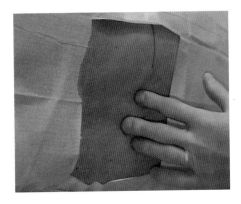

Infiltrate the deeper tissues with local anaesthetic.

- Use the local anaesthetic needle to find the location and direction of the interspace.
- However, be cautious in thin patients, a 3 cm needle could conceivably penetrate the dura mater – in which case you would be giving the patient a spinal anaesthetic.
- This procedure does not have to hurt so if your patient is in pain you are doing something wrong. Lidocaine needs to be in the right place and have time to work.

Angle the spinal needle slightly towards the head and advance it through the skin and interspinous ligaments. Increased resistance may be felt passing through the ligamentum flavum.

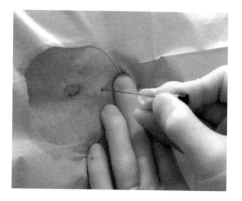

- You may feel the needle 'give' or even hear a 'click' as the dura is punctured.
- The 'feel' of the needle will be increased if the blunter Whitaker or Sprotte needle is used compared to the traditional Quincke cutting needle.

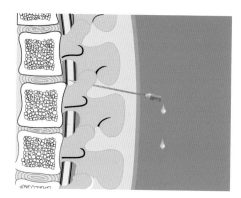

Remove the stilette and measure CSF pressure using a manometer set.

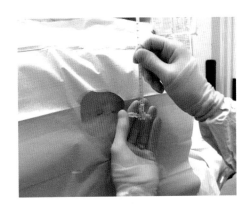

- If this is not available you could use an electronic pressure transducer set similar to that for measuring central venous pressure (CVP) or invasive arterial pressure.

Now collect the required CSF, then replace the stilette prior to removing the needle.

- If CSF does not flow, try rotating the needle through 90, 180° or 270° as it may be obstructed by a nerve root or flap of dura.
- If this fails, ask the patient to cough or to perform a Valsalva manoeuvre.
- Finally, you can ask an assistant to press intermittently on the patient's abdomen to increase CSF pressure.

Detach the manometer and collect the required CSF, usually into three numbered bottles.

- Number your specimen bottles. A falling red blood cell count from bottle one to bottle three suggests that there has been bleeding from the lumbar puncture itself rather than intrinsic bleeding within the CSF.

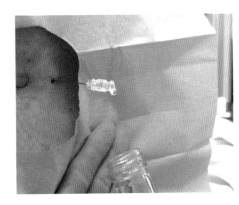

I Venous   II Arterial   III Central Venous   IV Airway   V Thoracic   VI Others   VII Supplemental Skills

Apply a dressing.

● Warn patients about post-dural puncture headache and tell them to report it if it develops.

● Prophylactic bed rest following lumbar puncture is of no benefit and should not be recommended anymore. It may increase the risk of venous thrombosis.

● Treat post-dural puncture headache with:
  ○ Bed rest
  ○ Simple analgesia
  ○ Rehydration – put up a drip and encourage oral fluids
  ○ Caffeine and antimigraine medication
  ○ If persistent, get an anaesthetist involved who might consider performing epidural blood patch.

27. Nasogastric Tube Insertion

Position the subject sitting up and explain what you are going to do.

Consider using topical lidocaine spray to anaesthetize the nose.

- Identify which is the most patent nostril by asking the patient to sniff through each nostril in turn.
- Ask about previous surgery or trauma to the nose or previous failed attempts at tube insertion.
- Local anaesthetic spray takes some time to have any effect. This is an uncomfortable procedure so give the spray some time to work.

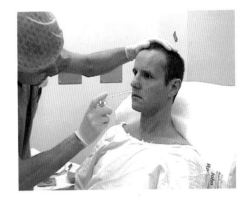

Lubricate the tube with lidocaine gel, then insert the tube parallel to the floor of the nose.

- You can insert the lidocaine gel in the nose then pass the tube through it.
- Gentle, sustained pressure, with a slight rotating movement, is the most effective method of getting the nasogastric tube (NG) through the nose. Do not force the tube or you will cause epistaxis.
- If you meet resistance, do not force it – try the other nostril.
- If the tube keeps coiling up in the mouth, use a new NG tube which has been kept in the fridge to make it more rigid.

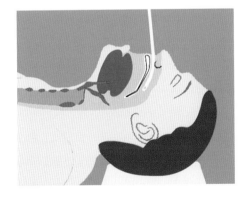

When the tube reaches the oropharynx ask the subject to swallow.

- Give the patient a drink of water and ask them to take small sips.
- If the patient coughs the NG tube may be entering the larynx, so withdraw a little and allow the patient to settle.

I Venous   II Arterial   III Central Venous   IV Airway   V Thoracic   VI Others   VII Supplemental Skills

- Flexing the neck should help to prevent the tube entering the larynx.

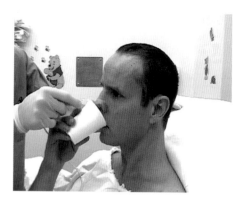

Ask the subject to keep swallowing as you advance the tube down the oesophagus. Correct placement can be confirmed by aspiration of gastric contents.

- Gastric contents may be bile-stained. If there is any doubt, check the pH of the aspirated liquid.

- Listen over the stomach whilst injecting air. Loud bubbling is very suggestive of gastric placement but not absolute.

- It is policy in some institutions that any NG tube intended for feeding must have position confirmed by X-ray prior to commencing feed.

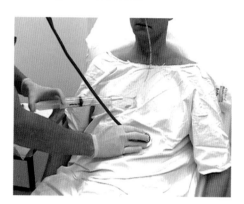

Connect a collection bag and tape the tube in position.

- The tube must be securely taped in place. Very occasionally, it will need to be sutured, for example after oesophageal or oropharyngeal surgery when re-insertion may be hazardous.

- The nares can develop pressure necrosis if the nasogastric (NG) tube is taped too tightly in place.

- Prolonged NG tube usage is associated with the development of sinusitis.

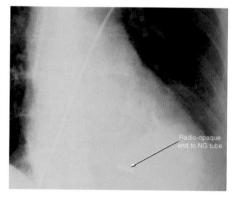

Radio-opaque
end to NG tube

In an unconscious patient, there are several tips and tricks to successful NG tube placement:

- Splitting a nasopharyngeal airway along its length, inserting it into the nose then inserting the NG tube through this. The split nasopharyngeal airway can then be removed over the NG tube.

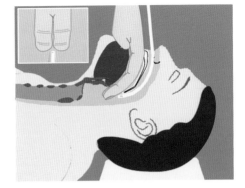

- Perform direct laryngoscopy, then use Magill forceps to direct the NG tube behind the larynx into the oesophagus.
- Using two fingers of your left hand to elevate the larynx, then advance the NG tube along the fingers.

Venous   II Arterial   III Central Venous   IV Airway   V Thoracic   VI Others   VII Supplemental Skills

28. Male Catheterisation

Position the patient supine.

- This can be stressful so ensure noise and interruptions are kept to a minimum.

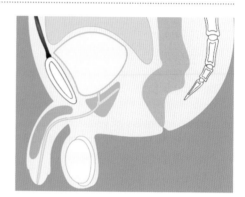

Thoroughly wash the area with water-based antiseptic solution. Repeat with fresh solution.

- Keep one hand 'clean' and use the other to hold the penis. Your 'clean' hand will be the one which you introduce the catheter with.

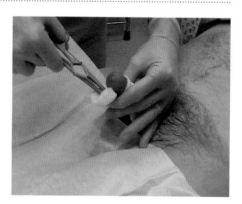

Pick up the penis with a sterile swab and withdraw the foreskin (if present).

Position the sterile drape. Thoroughly clean the glans penis with antiseptic solution (some patients will require more cleaning than others!).

Instil local anaesthetic gel down the penis and gently pinch the tip of the glans penis to prevent reflux. Allow time for the local anaesthetic gel to take effect.

- Inject the lidocaine gel slowly as it will be painful if you are too forceful.
- Massage the ventral surface of the penis with the local anaesthetic syringe to spread the gel and give it more time to work.

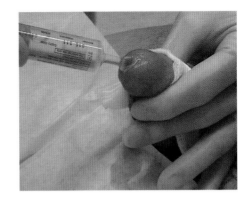

Pick up the catheter with a second clean pair of forceps then pass it along the penis to its full extent.

- If resistance is met it may help to apply gentle traction to the penis.
- Alternatively use a catheter with a coudé tip.
- If all this fails, a finger inserted rectally can help to get the catheter through the prostate.

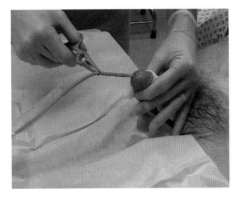

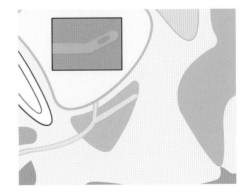

Fill the catheter balloon to its required volume with sterile water or saline.

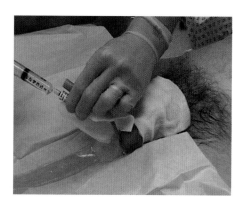

Withdraw the catheter until you meet resistance when the catheter balloon is at the bladder neck.

● There should be no initial resistance to this withdrawal – if there is, it suggests that you have inflated the balloon in the urethra. Deflate the balloon, withdraw the catheter and start again.

● If you have retracted the foreskin, you *must* pull it forward to prevent subsequent paraphimosis.

Finish by connecting the drainage system.

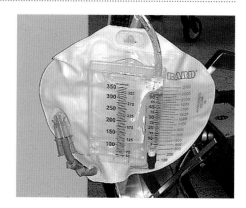

29. Female Catheterisation

Get help to lift the legs carefully and synchronously.

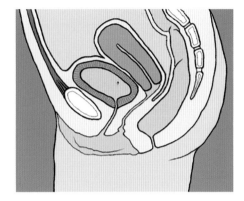

- This needs to be done with sensitivity in awake patients and you should consider having a chaperone with you.
- Extra care is needed in patients with hip or knee replacements.
- In unconscious patients placing the soles of the feet together helps to hold them in position.

Thoroughly clean the area with water-based antiseptic, then repeat with fresh solution.

- Ensure your equipment is complete and within reach.
- Keep one hand 'clean' and use the other to hold open the labia. The 'clean' hand will be the one which you introduce the catheter with.

Separate the labia to clean the vulva thoroughly.

- Part the labia with two fingers of one hand.
- Move your swab from anterior to posterior as the rectum is relatively more 'dirty'.

Position the sterile drape.

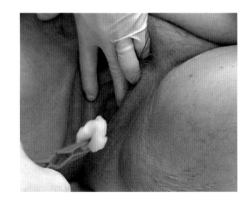

Pick up the catheter with clean forceps and insert it into the urethral orifice.

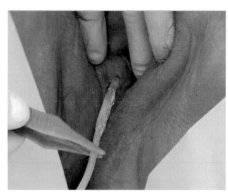

- This can be more difficult than you might expect particularly in obese patients – the urethra is sometimes hidden in mucosal folds or may lie further up the vagina.
- If in doubt identify the clitoris, then go posteriorly in the midline until you see the urethral opening.
- If you end up catheterising the vagina it may help to leave that catheter *in situ* whilst you try again with another to avoid making the same mistake twice.
- A small amount of lidocaine gel may assist urethral insertion.

Connect the collection bag immediately to prevent urine spillage.

Fill the catheter balloon to its required volume with sterile water.

Finally withdraw the catheter until resistance is met at the bladder neck.

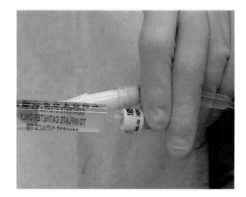

- There should be no resistance to this initial withdrawal – if there is, deflate the balloon, withdraw the catheter and start again.

30. Suprapubic Catheterisation

You should be supervised doing this procedure before doing it for the first time on your own. However, there may be circumstances when there is no other option other than for you to do it.

Ensure the bladder is full before you start. Percuss and palpate the position of the distended bladder in the midline.

- If you cannot manually feel the bladder, you should not proceed.
- Place absorbent pads or towels under the patient before you start – it may be messy!

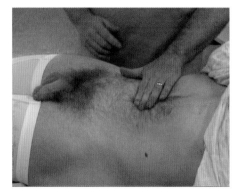

Shave excess hair and then wash hands prior to putting on sterile gloves and prepping the skin.

Infiltrate the skin over the bladder with local anaesthetic. Then infiltrate deeper tissues down to the bladder.

- Aim to locate the bladder and aspirate urine during this process. This will give you a good idea how deep the bladder is situated under the skin.

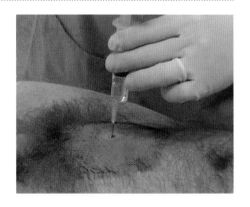

Incise the skin and deep tissues in the midline with a scalpel blade.

- There should be no major bleeding if you stay in the midline, but the inferior epigastric vessels lie just either side of the midline.

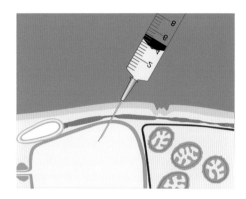

Insert the introducing sheath with the trocar, then remove the trocar and rapidly introduce the catheter.

- You may need to use a twisting motion to get the trocar through the tissues into the bladder.
- Once the trocar is removed, work quickly as the bladder will empty out of the sheath rapidly.

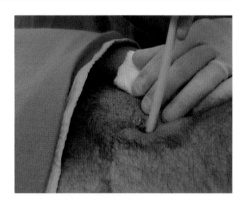

Fill the catheter balloon and connect to a catheter bag.

- Use the correct volume of water to fill the catheter balloon, it may not be you who removes the catheter.

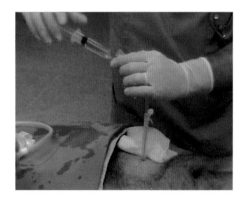

I Venous   II Arterial   III Central Venous   IV Airway   V Thoracic   VI Others   VII Supplemental Skills

Remove the introducing sheath by tearing
along the seam. Pull the balloon up to the
bladder wall, then apply a dressing over
the skin insertion point.

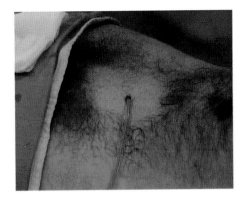

31. Knee Aspiration

Position the patient supine with the knee extended.

- Joint aspiration (arthrocentesis) should always be performed to make the diagnosis in unexplained mono-arthritis.

- Successful performance of this procedure requires knowledge of the anatomy of the knee. Otherwise the procedure will be considerably more painful and difficult.

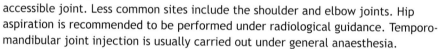

- Arthrocentesis may be performed on many joints. Knee aspiration is the most commonly performed and accessible joint. Less common sites include the shoulder and elbow joints. Hip aspiration is recommended to be performed under radiological guidance. Temporo-mandibular joint injection is usually carried out under general anaesthesia.

Widely prep the area.

- Strict aseptic technique is essential.

Palpate the supero-lateral aspect of the patella. Mark the skin one fingerbreadth above and one fingerbreadth lateral to this site.

- Both lateral and medial approaches are described, although the lateral approach is now more common.

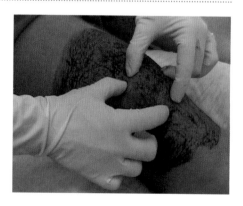

After infiltrating the skin with lidocaine using a 23G needle, infiltrate the deeper tissues with an 21G needle.

Direct the needle at 45° infero-medially, under the patella.

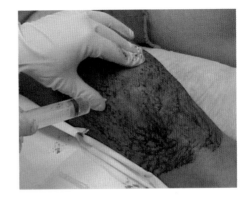

Insert the needle to 2-4 cm depth. Then aspirate, the syringe should fill with fluid.

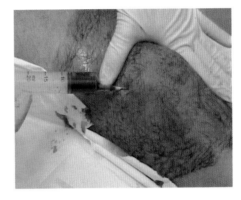

- Use the non-dominant hand to compress the opposite side of the joint or the patella which should help you to complete the joint aspiration.

- As the knee joint empties of fluid, the joint surfaces will all be brought closer together. Be careful that your needle tip does not cause trauma to the opposite joint surfaces in this way.

- If you need to give intra-articular steroids immediately following aspiration of fluid, place a clip or haemostat on the hub of the needle. With the needle thus stabilised, the fluid syringe can be disconnected and the fluid sent for studies. The steroid-filled syringe can then be attached to the needle and the injection administered.

When complete remove the needle and apply a dressing.

I Venous   II Arterial   III Central Venous   IV Airway   V Thoracic   VI Others   VII Supplemental Skills

VII
Supplemental Skills Section

I Venous

II Arterial

III Central Venous

IV Airway

V Thoracic

VI Others

VII Supplemental Skills

32. Emergencies

Emergencies may arise *de novo* at any time, for example:

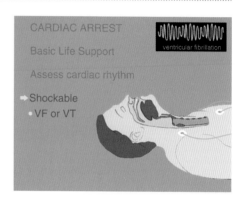

- Ventricular fibrillation secondary to myocardial ischaemia.
- Cardiovascular collapse due to septicaemia or pulmonary embolus.

They may result from trauma or in the post-operative period, for example:

- Major haemorrhage.
- Airway obstruction.

Or they may result from your own intervention, for example:

- Anaphylactic reaction to administered drugs.
- Tension pneumothorax after central line insertion.
- Hypoxia due to excessive sedation.

Many situations can be prevented from progressing to full cardiorespiratory arrest if potential precipitants are identified and rectified early. Before undertaking any intervention you must be proficient at dealing with the common complications and emergencies. These include:

Cardiorespiratory arrest

Anaphylaxis

Hypovolaemic shock

Tension pneumothorax

Major haemorrhage.

General Plan

1. **Recognise there is a problem.**

2. **Stop what you are doing.**

   - It may be the cause of the problem!

3. **Call for help – don't be proud.**

   - Immediately send anybody near you (nurse, porter or the patient's relative) to summon more senior help and the cardiac arrest/emergency trolley.

4. **A – Check the Airway is clear.**

   - Ask the patient if they are OK. If they answer then not only is their airway clear but their blood pressure must be perfusing their brain. Remove vomitus or foreign body from the mouth. Give oxygen by face mask at a flow rate of 10 l/min.

5. **B – Check for Breathing.**

   - Rapidly check for air movement, assess the patient's respiratory rate. Is chest expansion equal both sides?

6. **C – Check the Circulation.**

   - Feel for a central pulse – carotid or femoral. If you cannot feel one, start cardiopulmonary resuscitation immediately.

7. **Attach monitoring to the patient.**

   - Record baseline observations.

8. **Think about the underlying cause and how to treat it.**

   - By the time you have done all of these, the cavalry should be arriving. ...

I Venous   II Arterial   III Central Venous   IV Airway   V Thoracic   VI Others   VII Supplemental Skills

Anaphylaxis

True anaphylaxis is an immunoglobulin E (IgE) hypersensitivity reaction manifest as: dyspnoea, hypotension, angio-oedema and urticaria. Other features include abdominal symptoms of pain, nausea and vomiting as well as anxiety and rhinitis/conjunctivitis.

Possible allergens in clinical practice are:

1. Antibiotics – classically penicillin.
2. Parenteral vitamin supplements – usually the carrier solution that is allergenic.
3. Colloids – particularly gelatine-based products.
4. Contrast media used in radiology.
5. Muscle relaxants used in anaesthesia – particularly suxamethonium (scoline).
6. Patients may present after exposure to naturally occurring agents such as bee stings or peanuts.

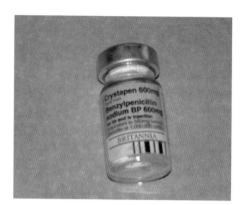

If a patient tells you they are allergic to a drug, ask them exactly what happened when they had the allergic reaction.

● For example, diarrhoea and vomiting after antibiotics is very unlikely to be true allergy, whereas a rash and wheeziness sounds more like it is allergenic.

A proven anaphylactic reaction should be followed up to identify the allergen.

● Following resuscitation (within 1 h of onset) send 10 ml clotted blood for mast cell tryptase assay and/or IgE analysis.
● Refer the patient to a specialist to determine the allergen.

Some patients claim to be allergic to local anaesthetic because they reacted with tachycardia and anxiety after a dental injection and the local 'didn't work'.

● Inadvertent injection of local anaesthetic containing adrenaline into a vessel is a more likely cause.

I Venous   II Arterial   III Central Venous   IV Airway   V Thoracic   VI Others   VII Supplemental Skills

Anaphylaxis management algorithm

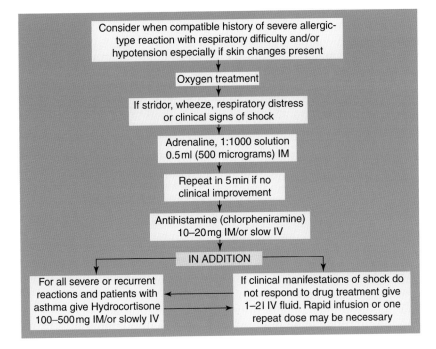

Consider when compatible history of severe allergic-type reaction with respiratory difficulty and/or hypotension especially if skin changes present

↓

Oxygen treatment

↓

If stridor, wheeze, respiratory distress or clinical signs of shock

↓

Adrenaline, 1:1000 solution 0.5 ml (500 micrograms) IM

↓

Repeat in 5 min if no clinical improvement

↓

Antihistamine (chlorpheniramine) 10–20 mg IM/or slow IV

↓

IN ADDITION

For all severe or recurrent reactions and patients with asthma give Hydrocortisone 100–500 mg IM/or slowly IV

If clinical manifestations of shock do not respond to drug treatment give 1–2 l IV fluid. Rapid infusion or one repeat dose may be necessary

- An inhaled beta2-agonist such as salbutamol may be used if bronchospasm does not respond rapidly to other treatment.

- If profound shock is judged to be immediately life threatening give CPR if necessary. Consider giving adrenaline 1:10 000 in 1 ml increments.

- Crystalloids may be safer than colloid which have a 1:10 000 incidence of anaphylactoid reactions.

Adult Basic Life Support

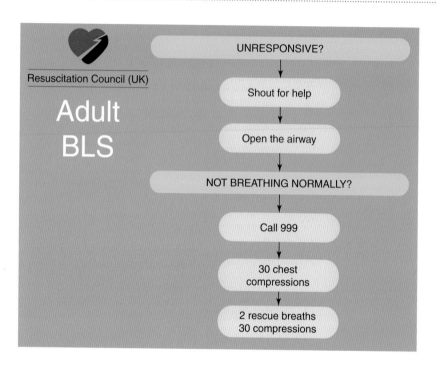

1. Make sure the victim, any bystanders, and you are safe.
2. Diagnose cardiac arrest if a victim is unresponsive and not breathing normally.

- Check the victim for a response.
- Gently shake the victim's shoulders and ask loudly, 'Are you all right?'

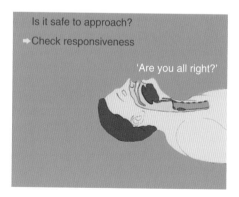

3. If they respond, leave them in the position in which you find them (provided there is no further danger).

- Try to find out what is wrong and get help if needed.
- Reassess regularly.

4. If the patient does not respond, shout for help, turn the victim supine and open the airway using head tilt/chin lift (see Basic Airway section).

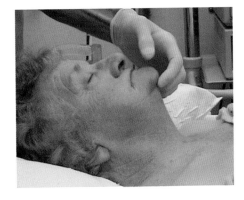

5. Keeping the airway open, look, listen and feel for normal breathing.

- Look – for chest movement.
- Listen – at the victim's mouth for breath sounds.
- Feel – for air on your cheek.
- In the first few minutes after cardiac arrest, a victim may be barely breathing, or taking infrequent, noisy, agonal gasps which are not to be confused with normal breathing.

6. If the victim is breathing normally, put them into the recovery position and send for help, or call for an ambulance.

- Keep checking for continued breathing.

7. If the victim is not breathing normally, call for an ambulance (you may need to leave the victim and go yourself). Start chest compressions:

- Kneel by the side of the victim, place the heel of one hand in the centre of the victim's chest, then the heel of your other hand on top of the first hand. Interlock your fingers and apply pressure to the centre of the chest.

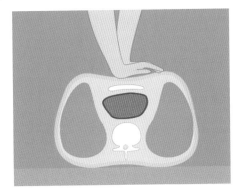

- Position yourself vertically above the victim's chest and, with your arms straight, press down on the sternum 4-5 cm.
- After each compression, release all the pressure on the chest without losing contact between your hands and the sternum. Repeat 100 times a minute, with compression and release taking an equal amount of time.

8. Combine chest compression with rescue breathing.

- After 30 compressions open the airway using head tilt and chin lift.
- Pinch the victim's nose closed, let the mouth open, but maintain chin lift.
- Blow into the victim's mouth over one second whilst watching the chest rise.
- Maintaining airway position, take your mouth away and watch for the chest to fall as air comes out.
- Blow into the victim's mouth once more to give a total of two effective rescue breaths. Then return your hands without delay to the sternum and give 30 further chest compressions. Continue with chest compressions and rescue breaths in a 30:2 ratio.
- Only interrupt resuscitation if the victim starts breathing normally.
- If you are not able, or willing, to give rescue breaths, give chest compressions only at 100 a minute.

9. Continue resuscitation until qualified help arrives and takes over, the victim starts breathing normally, or you become exhausted.

Adult Advanced Life Support

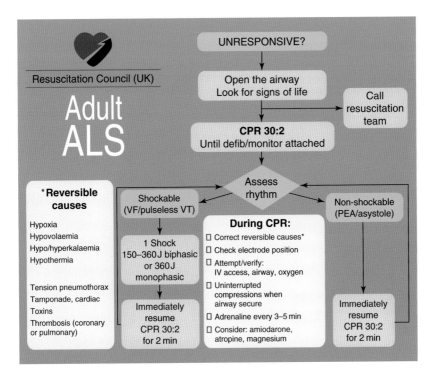

The fundamental basis of ALS is to maintain the circulation whilst distinguishing shockable arrhythmias such as *ventricular fibrillation (VF)* or *ventricular tachycardia (VT)* – from *asystole* which may respond to anticholinergic medication, and *pulseless electrical activity (PEA)* which often has an underlying cause.

Survival following cardiac arrest with asystole or PEA is unlikely unless a reversible cause can be found and treated effectively. So, when presented with a patient with electrical activity but no cardiac output, mentally run through all the reversible causes of PEA as this is the patient's only chance of survival.

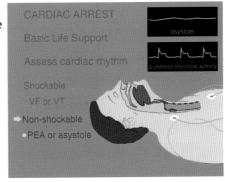

- **H**ypoxia
- **H**ypovolaemia
- **H**yperkalaemia, hypokalaemia, hypocalcaemia, acidaemia and other metabolic disorders
- **H**ypothermia
- **T**ension pneumothorax

- Tamponade
- Toxic substances
- Thromboembolism (pulmonary embolus/coronary thrombosis).

Treat ventricular fibrillation/pulseless ventricular tachycardia (VF/VT) with a single shock, followed by immediate resumption of CPR (30:2 ratio).

- Do not reassess the rhythm or feel for a pulse. After 2 min of CPR, check the rhythm and give another shock (if indicated).

The recommended initial energy for biphasic defibrillators is 150-200 J. Give second and subsequent shocks at 150-360 J.

- The recommended energy when using a monophasic defibrillator is 360 J for both the initial and subsequent shocks.
- If there is doubt about whether the rhythm is asystole or fine VF, do *not* attempt defibrillation; instead, continue chest compression and ventilation.

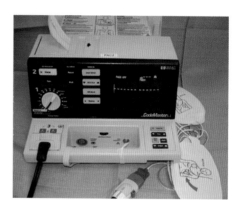

Adrenaline is still used in human resuscitation, despite there being no direct human evidence of it increasing survival. The alpha-adrenergic actions of adrenaline cause vasoconstriction, which increases myocardial and cerebral perfusion pressure during cardiac arrest.

- For VF/VT, give adrenaline 1 mg IV if VF/VT persists after a second shock.
- Repeat the adrenaline every 3-5 min thereafter if VF/VT persists.
- For PEA/asystole, give adrenaline 1 mg IV as soon as IV access is achieved and repeat every 3-5 min.

Other antiarrhythmic drugs used include amiodarone and lidocaine.

- If VF/VT persists after three shocks, give amiodarone 300 mg by bolus injection. A further 150 mg may be given for recurrent or refractory VF/VT, followed by an infusion of 900 mg over 24 h.
- If amiodarone is not available, lidocaine 1 mg kg^{-1} may be used instead.

Provide artificial ventilation as soon as possible. Expired air ventilation (rescue breathing) is effective but as expired oxygen concentration is only 16–17%, ventilation with oxygen-enriched air should commence as soon as possible.

- Some pocket resuscitation masks, which enable mouth-to-mask ventilation, allow supplemental oxygen to be given.
- Use a two-hand technique to maximise the seal with the patient's face.

Once an airway device has been inserted, ventilate the lungs at a rate of about 10 breaths per minute and continue chest compression without pausing during ventilation.

1. *Laryngeal mask airway (LMA)*: It is easy to insert, and ventilation using an LMA is more efficient and easier than with a bag-mask. Although an LMA does not protect the airway as reliably as a tracheal tube, pulmonary aspiration is uncommon when using an LMA during cardiac arrest.

2. *Combitube*: It is relatively easy to insert and ventilation is more efficient and easier than with a bag-mask. However, ensure you do not ventilate the wrong port of the Combitube.

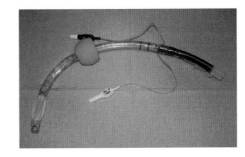

3. *Endotracheal intubation*: It is the optimal method of maintaining the airway during CPR. You must assess whether the tube is in the trachea:

- Primary assessment should include bilateral observation of chest expansion, bilateral auscultation in the axillae (breath sounds equal and adequate), and auscultation over the epigastrium (no breath sounds).

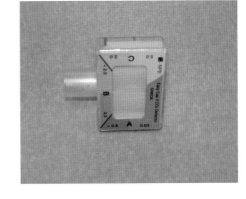

- Secondary confirmation of tracheal tube placement by an exhaled CO_2 or oesophageal detector device should reduce the risk of unrecognised oesophageal intubation. If there is doubt about correct tube placement, look directly with a laryngoscope to see if the tube is through the vocal cords.

During cardiac arrest, pulmonary blood flow may be so low that there is insufficient exhaled CO_2 to be detected.

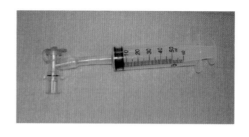

- If exhaled CO_2 is detected during cardiac arrest it indicates reliably that the tube is in the trachea or a main bronchus.

- If no exhaled CO_2 is detected , tracheal tube placement can be confirmed with an oesophageal detector device. Connect the device to the endotracheal tube and rapidly withdraw the plunger. If aspiration of air is difficult the tube is likely to be in the oesophagus.

4. *Cricothyroidotomy*: If an apnoeic patient cannot be ventilated with a bag-mask, or an endotracheal tube or alternative airway device cannot be passed, a surgical or needle cricothyroidotomy may be lifesaving.

Peripheral venous cannulation is quicker, easier to perform and safer than central venous access.

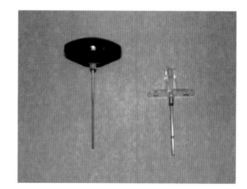

- Drugs injected peripherally must be followed by a flush of at least 20 ml of fluid.

- Central venous line insertion must cause minimal interruption of chest compression.

- If IV access is impossible, consider the intraosseous route for both children and adults which enables withdrawal of marrow for venous blood gas analysis, measurement of electrolytes and haemoglobin concentration.

- If intravenous or intraosseous access cannot be established, some drugs can be given by the tracheal route. The dose of adrenaline is 3 mg diluted to at least 10 ml with sterile water.

Consider giving other drugs during the resuscitation.

- Magnesium sulphate 8 mmol (4 ml of a 50% solution) for refractory VF, ventricular tachyarrhythmias; torsade de pointes; digoxin toxicity.

- Sodium bicarbonate (50 mmol) if cardiac arrest is associated with hyperkalaemia or tricyclic antidepressant overdose.

- Atropine 3 mg IV to block activity at both the sinoatrial (SA) node and the atrioventricular (AV) node which may increase sinus automaticity and facilitate AV node conduction.
- Calcium chloride 10%, 10 ml (6.8 mmol Ca^{2+}) is indicated during resuscitation from PEA if it is caused by hyperkalaemia; hypocalcaemia; calcium-channel-blocking drugs overdose and magnesium overdose (e.g. during treatment of pre-eclampsia).

Avoid giving calcium solutions and sodium bicarbonate simultaneously by the same venous route.

- Insoluble calcium carbonate may precipitate.
- Both these solutions cause extensive tissue damage if they extravasate.

33. Local Anaesthesia

Always use local anaesthesia (LA) when performing invasive medical procedures (with the possible exception of during lifesaving emergencies).

● As well as being kinder to your patients, it will improve your success rate by reducing the reflex withdrawal to pain.

● Patients in pain become anxious, agitated, sweaty and sometimes uncooperative.

Local anaesthetic drugs work by blocking fast sodium channels in nerve axons. This prevents the propagation of the nerve impulse along the axon.

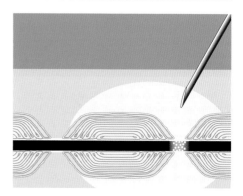

● Pain nerves are small, non-myelinated fibres that are blocked faster than large, myelinated fibres carrying touch, proprioception and motor power.

Local anaesthetics may be administered topically. Examples include: EMLA® and Ametop® creams for cutaneous analgesia; lidocaine gel for urinary catheterisation; lidocaine spray for pharyngeal analgesia and cocaine paste for nasopharyngeal analgesia.

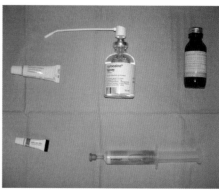

● EMLA and Ametop are not effective in all patients. They should not be applied to broken skin, mucous membranes or around the eyes.

● Topical anaesthesia of mucous membranes of the oropharynx is more effective if saliva production is reduced with an anticholinergic premedication, glycopyrrolate, for example 200 μg IV is appropriate.

Local anaesthetics may also be administered parenterally, given intravenously, intradermally, subcutaneously or intramuscularly depending on the drug and the circumstances.

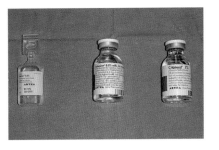

Local anaesthetic drugs are less effective in infected tissues.

- The injection is more painful.
- It can spread the infection.
- The lower pH of infected tissue slows passage of the drug through membranes.
- The increased vascularity of infected tissues increases systemic absorption of local anaesthetic drugs.

Avoid using adrenaline-containing local anaesthetic agents in tissues supplied by end-arteries – digits or the penis.

- The vasoconstriction may lead to distal ischaemia and necrosis.

Local anaesthetic drugs are toxic to the cardiovascular system (arrhythmias) and the central nervous system (seizures).

- Know the maximum safe limits for local anaesthetic agents in mg/kg.
- Choose the local anaesthetic agent and the concentration, then work out the maximum dose for this patient based on their weight. Then you can calculate the maximum volume of solution you can administer.
- An optical isomer of bupivacaine is available – levobupivacaine – which is 'safer' in terms of being less cardiotoxic than bupivacaine.

You MUST know how much local anaesthetic you are giving

Remember that 1 ml of a 1% solution contains 10 mg of the drug (it is 1 % of 1g per ml)

Calculate the dose you are giving before you start

I Venous   II Arterial   III Central Venous   IV Airway   V Thoracic   VI Others   VII Supplemental Skills

The onset of anaesthetic effect is variable – intradermal injection produces immediate analgesia whereas subcutaneous or intramuscular injection takes 2–3 min for effect.

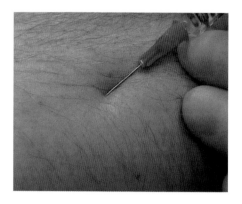

- Avoid testing the area for anaesthesia before the local anaesthetic has had a chance to work. Your patient may lose confidence if you test too soon and they can still feel something.

Duration of action is also variable – depending on the drug used; the vascularity of the site and the dose administered.

- For example lidocaine anaesthesia lasts for an hour or so, whereas bupivacaine usually gives several hours analgesia.

Avoid intravascular injection of local anaesthetic.

- Aspirate gently every time you move the needle and before you inject.
- Be aware that aspiration itself can move the needle tip.
- Alternatively, keep the needle moving during infiltration which will reduce the risk of significant intravascular injection.

I Venous   II Arterial   III Central Venous   IV Airway   V Thoracic   VI Others   VII Supplemental Skills

34. Monitoring

Monitoring may be invasive (breaches the skin) or non-invasive.

- Invasive monitoring is usually more accurate but is more prone to complications and misinterpretation.

Examples of situations to use monitoring:

- Pulse oximetry when sedative drugs have been used.
- ECG during central venous line insertion when the Seldinger wire may precipitate cardiac arrhythmias.
- Any procedure when you may be too pre-occupied to observe the patient fully.

Electrocardiography

The conducting system of the heart depolarise and repolarise during the cardiac cycle generating an electrical current, approximately 1–2 mV, which may be detected at the skin surface, amplified and converted to a visible format.

Always apply new electrodes, if you have to move one, use a fresh electrode.

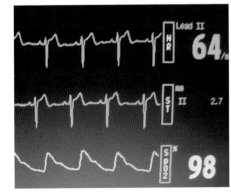

- Positioning one electrode at the apex of the heart and the others over the humeral heads usually works well.
- Contact and therefore signal strength can be improved by cleaning the skin by light abrasion and/or alcohol wipes.

Change the designated lead at the monitor to get the best QRS pattern.

- A large T wave can be counted by the monitor as a QRS complex and this will be displayed as double the actual heart rate.

The ECG monitor is electrically isolated and not earthed to prevent the risk of micro shock which could occur in a patient with central venous access.

● Never use faulty electrical equipment in contact with a patient.

The ECG can be used to guide correct placement of central lines and during pericardiocentesis.

● During central line placement, the appearance of ectopic beats on the ECG can indicate that the wire has entered the right atrium.

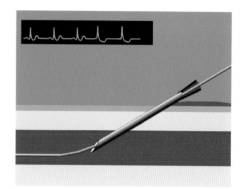

Non-invasive blood pressure

Wrap the blood pressure cuff around the upper arm and inflate whilst palpating the brachial pulse until the pulse disappears (up to 250 mmHg).

● This gives a guide to the systolic pressure and avoids the problem of the true systolic being missed in very hypertensive patients.

● Deflate the cuff completely before use, and then wrap it snugly (but not tightly) around the arm.

● Keep the cuff as proximal as possible which will minimise interference if the patient bends the arm.

● Keep the cuff approximately at heart level.

Now deflate the cuff slowly whilst listening with a stethoscope over the brachial artery releasing the pressure at about 2 mmHg/s.

● The sounds of turbulent flow as blood re-enters the artery are heard with two characteristic peaks (Korotkoff sounds).

● The systolic pressure corresponds to the first appearance of tapping sounds (I).

● The diastolic pressure corresponds to when the sound starts to fade (IV).

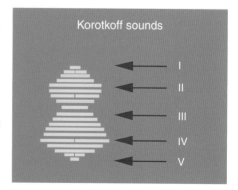

Korotkoff sounds

I
II
III
IV
V

Use the correct cuff size – the cuff width should be approximately half the circumference of the limb. If you use a cuff that is too small it may lead to over-estimation of the blood pressure.

- The precise algorithm used for measuring and calculating blood pressure used by automated non-invasive machines varies according to the manufacturer.

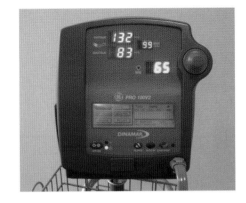

Avoid using NIBP on a limb with an intravenous infusion running as it can cause 'backing up' of the drip.

- If you have to do this, enclose the IV drip tubing within the blood pressure cuff – then when the blood pressure cuff is inflated, it will stop the drip backing up.

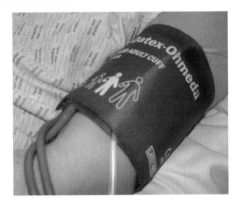

Pulse oximetry

A pulse oximeter gives a continuous measure of arterial oxygen saturation and pulse rate.

- There is a delay between the problem developing and the saturation falling so you need to respond quickly to any fall in saturation.

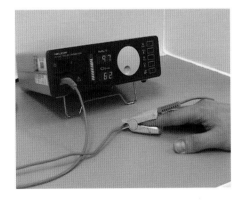

I Venous   II Arterial   III Central Venous   IV Airway   V Thoracic   VI Others   **VII Supplemental Skills**

The oxygen saturation of the blood is the percentage saturation of the population of haemoglobin molecules in a blood sample.

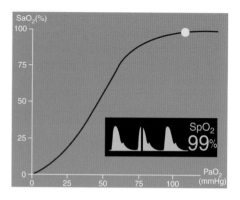

- In the lungs, where PaO_2 is high, oxygen binds readily to haemoglobin, but peripherally, where oxygen is needed for cell metabolism, the PaO_2 is low and therefore oxygen is released more easily.

A pulse oximeter works on the principle that oxyhaemaglobin and deoxyhaemoglobin absorb infrared (IR) lights to different degrees. Thus when an incident IR beam is passed through tissue the amount that is detected by a sensing electrode will depend on the relative amounts of oxy and deoxyhaemoglobin therefore giving the saturation.

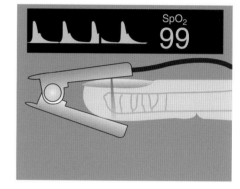

- Most oximeters also have an audible pulse tone, the pitch of which is proportional to the oxygen saturation – which is useful when one is not actually watching the monitor.

The algorithm used by the oximeter looks for a variable (pulsatile) signal and rejects all non-pulsatile components of the signal.

- Shivering can lead to inaccuracy as it causes the venous and capillary blood to appear 'pulsatile', along with other conditions causing pulsatile venous flow such as tricuspid regurgitation.

Select the probe you require and where it is going to go. The digit should be clean (remove nail varnish from that digit).

- Allow several seconds for the pulse oximeter to detect the pulse and calculate the oxygen saturation before trying an alternate site.

Look for a displayed pulsatile waveform.

- Without this, any reading is potentially misleading and should be ignored.

I Venous   II Arterial   III Central Venous   IV Airway   V Thoracic   VI Others   VII Supplemental Skills

Don't rely on the monitor – use your clinical judgement.

- Machines can be wrong; a normal saturation in an obviously cyanosed patient should not delay treatment.
- If the pulse oximeter is not detecting a pulse, it is not necessarily artefact, there may not be one and you should investigate and take prompt action.

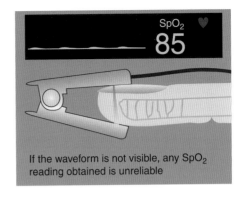

If the waveform is not visible, any SpO₂ reading obtained is unreliable

Invasive blood pressure measurement

Use invasive arterial pressure monitoring for:

- Patients on HDU or ICU who require continuous blood pressure measurement and multiple arterial blood sampling.
- Haemodynamically unstable patients undergoing surgery or treatment.
- Patients receiving vasoactive drugs.
- Where non-invasive blood pressure is not possible or inaccurate (e.g. during patient transfer).

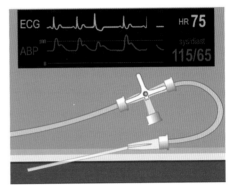

Preferentially use the radial artery to site the arterial line.

- Possible alternatives include: ulnar, femoral, dorsalis pedis or brachial arteries.
- Avoid the carotid artery – you could dislodge plaque precipitating a stroke.
- Avoid end-arteries or where there is distal ischaemia.

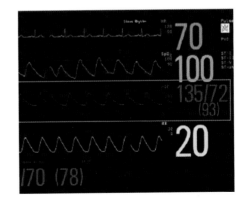

I Venous   II Arterial   III Central Venous   IV Airway   V Thoracic   VI Others   VII Supplemental Skills

I Venous   II Arterial   III Central Venous   IV Airway   V Thoracic   VI Others   VII Supplemental Skills

Check the arterial supply to the hand with the Allen test before the arterial line is inserted.

- Look for blanching or other signs of ischaemia and remove an arterial line if the hand is becoming ischaemic.
- Avoid siting the cannula where it will be kinked easily, for example the antecubital fossa.

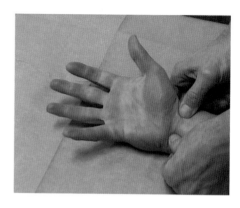

Zero the system and position the transducer at the horizontal level of the right atrium.

- Open the three way stopcock so that the transducer is open to the air (not the patient – as blood will start to come out of the three way tap under arterial pressure). The reading should then be zero.

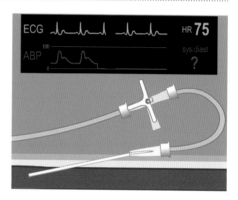

Be aware that the arterial waveform may 'flatten out' significantly after a period of time.

- First try moving the wrist as the tip of the cannula may be up against the vessel wall.
- It may be caused by thrombus beginning to form at the cannula tip which can be cleared by flushing.
- If the waveform is damped, the systolic and diastolic readings are inaccurate, but the mean blood pressure should still be accurate.

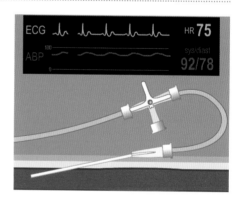

Central venous pressure measurement

The CVP may be measured using a direct transducer system as with the arterial line or with a manometer filled with intravenous fluid attached to the central venous catheter.

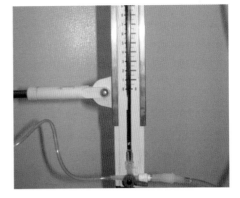

- The zero mark of the manometer needs to be positioned at the level of the right atrium, approximately the mid-axillary line in the 4th interspace in a supine patient.

Measurements should be taken in the same position each time using a spirit level and the zero point on the skin surface marked with a cross.

- Check that the catheter is not blocked or kinked and that intravenous fluid runs freely in, and blood freely out.
- Absolute CVP values are less important than trends. For example, an isolated CVP reading of $10\,cmH_2O$ is less useful than knowing the CVP has risen from 5 to $10\,cmH_2O$.

To measure the CVP, open the three-way tap so that the fluid from the bag fills the manometer tubing. Now turn the tap to open the lumen between patient and manometer.

- The fluid level will drop to the level of the CVP which is usually recorded in centimetres of water (cmH_2O).
- It will be slightly pulsatile and will continue to rise and fall slightly with breathing, record the average reading.

Alternatively, electronic transducers similar to those used for invasive arterial blood pressure measurement are often used in the operating theatres or the ICU to give a continuous readout of CVP along with a display of the waveform.

- The CVP reading from an electronic monitor is sometimes given in mmHg (same as blood pressure). The values can easily be converted knowing that $10\,cmH_2O$ is equivalent to 7.5 mmHg which is equivalent to 1 kPa.

I Venous   II Arterial   III Central Venous   IV Airway   V Thoracic   VI Others   VII Supplemental Skills

35. Oxygenation

Oxygen is supplied either by cylinders or from a central, piped supply to a wall outlet.

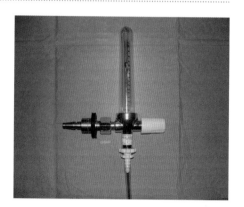

- For oxygen delivery by face mask, the gas first passes through a rotameter, which can be typically set at flows between 1 and 15 l/min.

- These rotameters are gas specific, so oxygen rotameters can only be connected to oxygen supplies.

- Valve regulators are alternatives to rotameters commonly found on cylinders and used as shown.

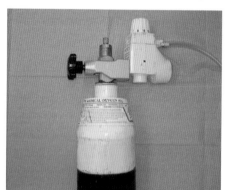

- In the UK, oxygen cylinders are black with white shoulders. This varies from country to country.

There are several different types of oxygen mask:

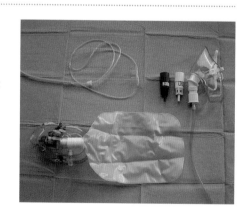

1. Basic Hudson mask delivers oxygen through a small adapter so the patient inhales a mixture of oxygen and room air. The inspired oxygen concentration varies depending on the peak inspiratory flow rate and the oxygen flow rate.

2. Venturi mask delivers a fixed oxygen concentration (24%, 28% or 35%) with the correct gas flow and are useful when a set level is required. Chronic obstructive pulmonary disease patients can be given 24% for example to avoid high-inspired concentrations.

3. Rebreathing (reservoir) masks can deliver greater than 80% inspired oxygen.

   Caution: These should be avoided when the patient may be exhaling toxic fumes (e.g. carbon monoxide from a house fire).

4. Nasal specula can be used in patients who are intolerant of face masks, but they deliver unpredictable concentrations of oxygen, depending on whether the patient is nasal- or mouth-breathing.

5. Anaesthetic face masks with Ambubag® are the only means of delivering 100% oxygen via a face mask The exhaled gases are vented and there is no entrainment of atmospheric air.

Reasons why a patient might need *more* than the 21% oxygen in atmosphere air include:

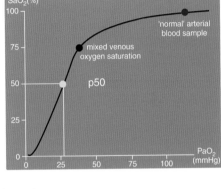

- Increased oxygen requirements – shivering, sepsis, raised metabolic rate, shock.

- Reduced alveolar ventilation – airway obstruction, sedative drugs, CNS disease, mechanical lung problems, increased alveolar deadspace.

- Reduced oxygen uptake from the lungs – shunt, pulmonary oedema, diffusion impairment.

- Reduced oxygen-carrying capacity of the blood – anaemia, carbon monoxide poisoning.

An important (but less obvious) reason to give supplemental oxygen to patients is to buy you time in an emergency.

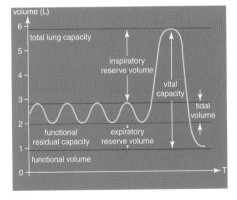

- The vital capacity is approximately 5-6 l in an adult. Breathing room air, the oxygen reserve in the lungs is $21\% \times 5 l = 1 l$. However breathing 60% oxygen, this is increased dramatically to 3 l, which can maintain oxygenation for longer.

- It is particularly important to provide supplemental oxygen if the patient is to be sedated as they may already be some way down the haemoglobin-oxygen dissociation curve.

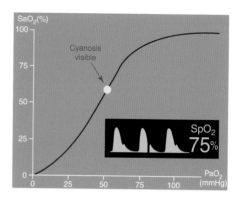

36. Sedation

Sedation is the use of a drug or drugs to depress the central nervous system enabling invasive treatment to be carried out.

Explain to the patient what you are going to do and obtain informed consent before administering any sedation.

- Your hospital should have guidelines for safe sedation practice which should be followed.
- A sympathetic and careful explanation to the patient of what is going to happen will help to reduce sedation requirements.
- You may require written informed consent, again depending on local policy.

Undertake a brief history and examination to exclude additional risk factors for sedation such as lung disease or neuromuscular conditions.

- Avoid sedating patients with chronic obstructive pulmonary disease or altered level of consciousness.

Check all required equipment. The patient should be on a tipping trolley with suction and resuscitation equipment close to hand. They should be fasted – ideally for a minimum of 4 h.

- There will be local guidelines for this at your hospital.

Monitor the patient. Administer oxygen by mask or nasal specs.

- Always have an assistant helping you. Not only may this person be useful to monitor the patient and get you equipment if required, they can act as the chaperone. There have been instances where sedated patients have accused medical practitioners of assault after being administered benzodiazepines or other sedatives.
- Pulse oximetry is the minimum acceptable monitoring. Blood pressure and ECG monitoring in addition would be ideal.
- Delegate a trained assistant to monitor the patient if you are going to be occupied with the invasive procedure.

Secure venous access

- A 22G cannula is fine. Avoid using a 'butterfly' needle as this can cut out of the vein easily.

Select the sedative drug carefully.

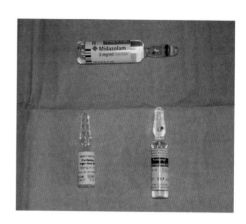

- Use a benzodiazepine such as midazolam if the patient is anxious. Use an opioid if the procedure will be painful even with judicious local anaesthesia.

- Do not use anaesthetic induction agents such as propofol or ketamine – their safety margin is narrower than that for opioids and benodiazepines.

- Entonox is an excellent analgesic sedative with a 'ceiling effect' as it has fixed composition of nitrous oxide: oxygen (50:50).

- The drugs and techniques used should carry a margin of safety wide enough to render sudden loss of consciousness unlikely.

- However, all sedative drugs, given in sufficient quantities, will render a patient unconscious – therefore administer the drugs in small aliquots rather than in large boluses.

Draw up the chosen sedative drug, and dilute if necessary, so that you can administer the drug accurately in increments.

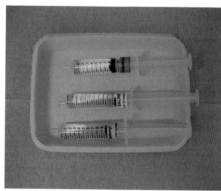

- For example, when using midazolam, draw up 10 mg in a 10 ml syringe and dilute with 0.9% normal saline such that the final concentration is 1 mg/ml. Label the syringe!

- Administer 0.5-1 ml of this solution at a time ($\times$ 0.5-1 mg aliquots), depending on the patient.

- Try to avoid polypharmacy as this is when the incidence of complications increases.

- However, if you elect to use a combination of an opioid with a benzodiazepine it is best to give the opioid first and then allow sufficient time to observe an effect before adding the benzodiazepine.

Administer the sedative drug in incremental doses allowing sufficient time to observe an effect.

- Individual patient response to sedative drugs can vary significantly.
- Ensure verbal contact is maintained throughout. A level of sedation to aim for is where the patient has their eyes closed but will open them and respond if you ask a question.

The situation can rapidly deteriorate if an overdose of sedative drugs is administered.

- If satisfactory sedation cannot be achieved seek the help of an anaesthetist rather than continue to give further doses of sedative drugs.
- Stop the invasive procedure immediately and call for some help.
- Administer oxygen, open the airway using Basic Airway manoeuvres.
- Consider giving a reversal agent.
- *If verbal responsiveness is lost the patient requires a level of care identical to that needed for general anaesthesia.*

Have reversal agents available to administer if the patient shows signs of overdose such as airway obstruction or loss of consciousness.

- Benzodiazepines may be reversed using flumazenil 100 µg boluses up to 500 µg.
- Opioids may be reversed using naloxone in increments of 100 µg.
- Be aware that the duration of action of reversal agents may be less than that of the sedative agent – therefore re-sedation could occur which is why recovery is important.

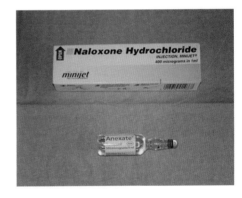

Observe the patient in a recovery area until they have recovered their normal mental status.

---

37. Sterile Technique

Four separate 'levels' of sterile technique are recognised:

1. 'Clean' – this involves hand-washing and the use of non-sterile, disposable gloves. Examples: body surface examination, venous cannulation, endotracheal intubation, nasogastric tube insertion.

2. 'Aseptic' – hand-washing using an evaporative solution such as chlorhexidine in alcohol followed by donning of sterile, disposable gloves using a sterile technique. Examples: arterial line insertion, long line insertion, urinary catheterisation.

3. 'Scrubbing up' for the operating theatre – a full 5-min 'scrub up'.

4. Sterile gown and glove – 3 min hand-washing followed by donning of sterile, disposable gown and sterile disposable gloves. Examples: central line insertion, chest drain insertion, lumbar puncture.

Aseptic donning of sterile gloves

Always wear gloves for patient contact and practical procedures.

- If you feel clumsy initially do not worry, you *will* get used to them.

Select an appropriate size and type of sterile glove.

- Avoid donning wet gloves, it will make it much harder to get the gloves on.

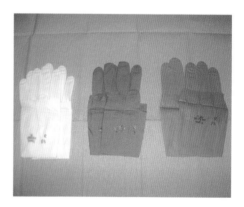

Wash and dry your hands or clean with alcohol solution and allow to dry.

- The bactericidal action only occurs following evaporation of the gel, so they must be allowed to dry before proceeding.

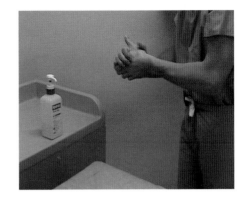

Open the gloves and put the first on touching only the inside surfaces

- Keep your hands 'high' at all times.
- Latex allergy to gloves can develop in medical staff. Some are simply allergic to the talcum powder. Latex- and talc-free products are readily available.

Now pick up the second glove, touching only the outside surface. Pull the glove onto the hand.

Now pull up the first glove taking care to only touch the outer surface.

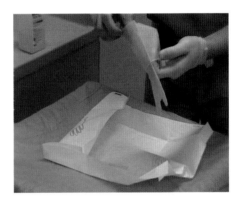

- Touch only the cuff of the glove with ungloved hand, and then only glove to glove for the other hand.
- Keep your hands clasped when you are not actually doing anything.

Always wash your hands after dealing with each patient.

- Inter-patient spread of infection by medical staff is a major cause of morbidity and mortality during a hospital stay.

Full surgical scrub

If you are going to 'scrub' for theatre, it needs to be for a full 5 min.
With your mask in place wet your arms to the elbow.

- Remember to put your mask on prior to starting your scrub.

I Venous   II Arterial   III Central Venous   IV Airway   V Thoracic   VI Others   VII Supplemental Skills

Apply scrub solution, wash both arms to the elbow and then rinse.

- Use aqueous iodine- or chlorhexidine-containing solutions as appropriate.
- Keep your elbows below your hands at all times so that contaminated water does not run down over your hands.

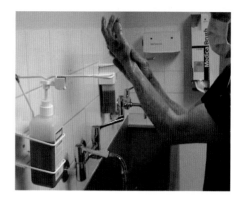

Take a scrub brush, clean beneath all nails.

- Use the enclose plastic pick to clean under the nails.

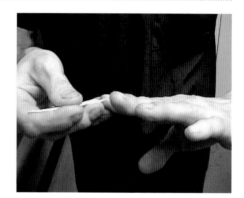

Scrub all nails and then each finger individually. Scrub both hands front and back. Scrub both arms to the elbow.

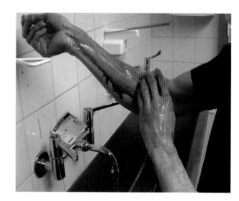

Rinse and then scrub both hands and arms again. Rinse for the final time and dry your hands.

- When drying, never bring the towel back over a clean area.

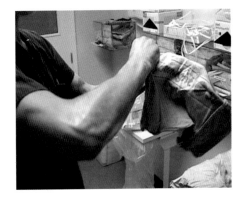

Lift and put on the gown touching only the interior surface of the collar and then arms.

- Get an assistant to tie up the back of the gown.

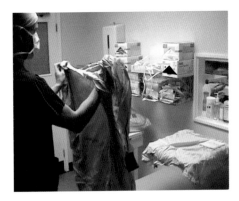

Put on the first glove touching only the interior leaving the cuff down.

Now put on the other glove touching only the exterior surface and pull it up the sleeve.

- Never let the fingers extend beyond the stockinette cuff during the procedure.
- Any contact with ungloved fingers constitutes contamination of the glove.

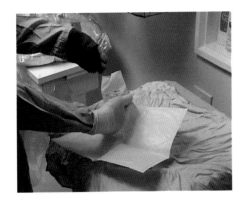

Finally pull up the first cuff touching only the exterior surface.

- Loose clothing can easily contaminate a sterile field so ensure ties, stethoscopes, etc. are not swinging free.

I Venous   II Arterial   III Central Venous   IV Airway   V Thoracic   VI Others   VII Supplemental Skills

Once you are 'sterile', keep your hands in sight and at waist level or above.

● If contamination occurs during either procedure, both gown and gloves must be discarded and new gown and gloves must be added.

Sterile gown and gloves

If you are scrubbing up in order to place a central line, it needs to be for at least 3 min.

● This is also suitable for aseptic procedures such as chest drain insertion and lumbar puncture.

With your mask in place wet your arms to the elbows.

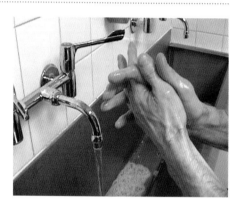

Apply scrub solution and wash both arms to the elbow and then rinse.

● Use aqueous iodine- or chlorhexidine-containing solutions as appropriate.
  ○ Apply more solution
  ○ Rub between fingers front and back
  ○ Interlock the fingers and scrub

Clean both thumbs.

- The thumbs are often missed out or neglected during scrubbing up.
  - Rub nails to palms.

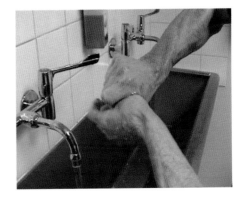

Finally rinse thoroughly and put on a gown as described earlier.

- Always keep your hands higher than your elbows so that dirty water from your arms does not run down over your clean hands.

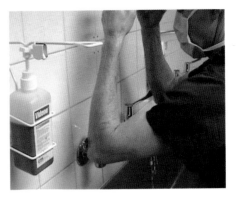

38. Suturing Techniques

First, think about whether there may be alternatives to suturing:

- Wound closure tapes (Steri-Strips®) are useful for very small wounds.
- Stainless steel staples are frequently used in wounds under high tension, including wounds on the scalp and trunk.
- Cyano-acrylate superglues are used to block pinpoint skin haemorrhages and to precisely appose wound edges.

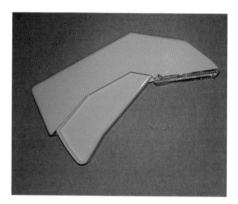

If you do need to suture, then select the appropriate suture for the wound you are closing:

- A *simple interrupted suture* has good tensile strength with low potential for causing wound oedema. It allows continual adjustment to align wound edges as the wound is sutured, but is slow and carries the risk of cross-hatched marks across the suture line.
- A *simple running suture* is useful for long wounds in which wound tension has been minimised with properly placed deep sutures and in which approximation of the wound edges is good.

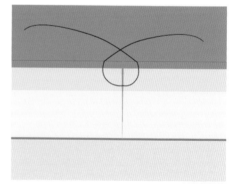

- A *running locked suture* is useful in wounds under moderate tension or in those requiring additional haemostasis because of oozing from the skin edges. They increase the risk of impaired microcirculation if placed too tightly.
- A *mattress suture* (vertical or horizontal) is useful in maximising wound eversion, reducing dead space and minimising tension across the wound.

- *Subcuticular suture* is useful in wounds with minimal tissue tension or dead space, and where the best possible cosmetic result is desired.

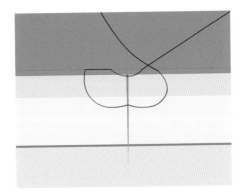

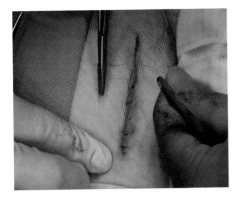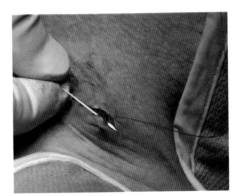

Then, think about what sort of suture material you need:

- Absorbable or non-absorbable – depending on how long the suture needs to retain its strength.
  - Use absorbable sutures in children to avoid the need for suture removal.
- Mono-filament or braided – depending on whether it needs to pass through tissues very smoothly.

Next, how thick does the suture material need to be?

- The strength of sutures varies according to the suture material and the diameter (gauge) of the suture.
- Suture gauge varies from 12/0 (ophthalmic sutures invisible to the naked eye) through 5/0 (0.1 mm diameter, used for skin suturing on the face) to 5 (almost 1 mm diameter), used to anchor drains.

I Venous   II Arterial   III Central Venous   IV Airway   V Thoracic   VI Others   **VII Supplemental Skills**

Finally think about what sort of needle you need. Suture needles are usually curved, and designed to be held in needle-holders. Straight needles, designed to be hand-held, carry an increased risk of accidental needlestick injury.

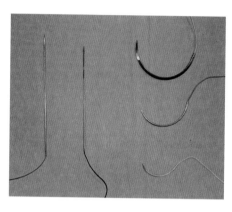

- *Atraumatic* (= round-bodied) needles are circular in cross-section and are used for suturing bowel, muscle, fascia and blood vessels.
- *Cutting* needles have a triangular body with a sharp edge on the inner curve of the needle that is directed towards the wound edge.
- *Reverse cutting* needles have a sharp edge on the outer curve of the needle that is directed away from the wound edge, which reduces the risk of the suture pulling through the tissue. Skin sutures tend to have reverse cutting needles for this reason.
- *Taper cut* needles share some of the features of round-bodied and cutting needles.

Always be generous with local anaesthesia if possible.

- A patient with a cut requiring suturing may well be in considerable discomfort already so use local anaesthesia.
- Try instilling local anaesthesia into the wound directly, then, after waiting for this to have some effect, injecting into the cut skin edges themselves.

Removal of sutures also requires thought:

- Sutures should not be removed too soon to prevent wound dehiscence.
- Non-absorbable sutures must be removed within 1-2 weeks of their placement, depending on the anatomic location.
- Prompt removal reduces the risk of suture marks, infection and tissue reaction. The average wound usually achieves approximately 8% of its expected tensile strength 1-2 weeks after surgery.
- The greater the tension across a wound, the longer the sutures should remain in place. As a guide, on the face, sutures should be removed in 5-7 days; on the neck, 7 days; on the scalp, 10 days; on the trunk and upper extremities, 10-14 days and on the lower extremities, 14-21 days.
- To remove a suture, elevate with forceps, and cut one side. Then, grasp the suture by the knot and gently pull towards the wound or suture line until it is completely removed.

Index